RUNNING FOR THE GLORY OF GOD

BOB JENNERICH

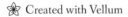

ALSO BY BOB JENNERICH

Get My Free Ebook: This Is God's Plan?! How We Can Be Certain in Days of Uncertainty

(You can download this book for free by going to my website BobJennerich.com)

- **Also Available on Amazon:**
- Facing Life's Challenges Head On
- God Is Everywhere! Recognizing Our Extraordinary God in Ordinary Life
- Don't Be A Hypocrite and Other Lessons I'm Still Learning from the Sermon on the Mount
- You can connect with me on Facebook at Facebook. com/BobJennerich, and Twitter.com/ bob_jennerich. Go to BobJennerich.com find a link to my other books. You can also subscribe to my newsletter at BobJennerich.com. I like to treat my newsletter subscribers well by giving discounts and freebies that I don't make available to the general public. I also like to talk to you! You can also read my blog and listen to sermons I preached at Grace Redeemer Community Church, Garland, TX.

CONTENTS

INTRODUCTION

I have been running my entire life. I practically came out of the womb running. Not distance running but running like kids run. Like Forrest Gump, if I was going anywhere, I was running! As a kid I played organized football, baseball, and basketball. The ball field was just a block from my house, and I would run there to play. I stopped growing in high school which made it hard to compete with my classmates in baseball, football, and basketball, so I joined the freshman cross-country team. Cross-country wasn't nearly as cool as being the star basketball player, but at my height, I had to accept reality. I was not born to play in the NBA.

For freshmen, the standard cross-country distance was two miles. The varsity course was 3.1 miles. Even if you're young and healthy, running that far still requires training. There's a difference between finishing and finishing well. In my years of running, I've passed plenty of runners who took off like they've been shot out of a cannon, only to be throwing up on the side of the road later in the race. Sadly, I've been that guy too! Distance running takes stamina, strategy, and pace. It's easy for most young and healthy people to train for a two or three-mile race, but learning strategy and pace takes a lifetime. Every race is different, especially since your physical condition changes as you age, and fitness can even fluctuate from day to day. Like most things in life, wisdom comes with time and experience.

I enjoyed the social aspect of being on the cross-country team. We only had a few boys on the freshman team. Most were friends whom I persuaded to join. Often high school basketball or baseball players would run cross-country to stay in shape. Most of my friends played other sports, and like me, didn't have any experience running cross-country. But we adapted quickly. I won the first four races in which I competed. Soon my friends surpassed me once they got into "cross-country" shape. That was ok though. Our rag-tag team of runners who played other sports turned out to be pretty good. We won the league championship that year.

I continued to run throughout high school. Cross-country in the fall, followed by winter track, then spring track. Winter track and spring track differed completely from cross-country. Cross-country is a single event race. Winter and spring track meets have a full slate of races ranging from 100 meters to two miles, plus relay races, and all the field events including pole vault, shot put, and javelin. The entire cross-country team, boys, girls, varsity, and freshmen totaled about 30 kids. Winter and spring track drew over 100 kids because of the variety of events, and because of the social aspect of these sports.

As I grew into my teenage years, I became a bit rebellious. It was more fun to figure out ways to avoid running than to actually run. I learned it was much easier to get lost in the crowd in winter and spring track than it was in cross-country. Our coach would run with us. There was no cutting corners because we were under his watchful eye and often running next to him. In winter and spring track, with over 100 kids practicing many different events, coaches couldn't keep track of everyone. I figured out that when the coach told us to go for a 5-mile run, we could run a half-mile to the ice cream parlor, chow down a fudge sundae, and then run back, and no one was the wiser.

Thus began my slide away from running, which is really the entire point of joining track, into trying to figure out how to avoid running. My ability to avoid running far exceeded my talent as a runner. My goals changed over my high school years. Running became a social event rather than a physical activity. The non-running part of track meets is a lot of fun. You board a bus with the team, hang out, laugh, and joke on your way to the meet. The meet lasts for hours, but your event is at most just a few minutes long. There's a ton of downtime, which is great for hanging out with friends, and especially trying to meet girls. I was much less interested in the running and much more interested in the opportunities that running provided.

My coaches got wise to me. Like most teenagers, I thought I had pulled the wool over everyone's eyes. I thought no one noticed my running avoidance. They probably let me get away with a lot because I just wasn't that talented. If the star of the team tried to pull the stuff I did, I'm sure there would have been greater repercussions. You can't have the star of the team leading everyone to the ice cream parlor for sundaes. For me there was only minor discipline. My punishment was that my coach always entered me in both the one-mile and two-mile races, the two longest races in the meet! My punishment for avoiding running: more running! It was cruel. They knew I had no chance to place in either race. It was straight up punishment.

If running was a punishment, I wanted to do it even less. Like when you punish your kids from not practicing the piano by making them practice the piano. It never has the desired effect. The cycle continued for me throughout high school. Enjoy the benefits of being on the track team but run as little as I could get away with.

When I graduated from high school, I assumed my running days were over. I went to college and then law school. My secular life included lots of parties, staying up late, getting up late, eating copious amounts of dining hall food, and being almost completely sedentary. I gained close to 30 pounds in college. After college, I went to law school in Michigan, where it's freezing cold most of the time. Next to the North Pole, Michigan was the least likely place to resurrect my running career. The partying and eating continued though I should have been studying. I packed on the weight. I once tipped the scale at 228 pounds, which is at least 60 pounds overweight for me.

It was the summer of 1992. I was disgusted with myself. I was extremely fat and couldn't climb a flight of stairs without gasping for air. With the encouragement of my then girlfriend Molly, who is now my wife of almost 30 years, I decided to do something about it. There was a track behind a school a block away from my apartment in Michigan. I tried to run one lap, a quarter mile. I couldn't make it. For someone who could run 10 miles in high school, that was a real wake-up call. I kept at it. I went back the next day and ran the full lap. Over the next few weeks, I increased to two laps, then three. Soon I could run a mile!

That encouraged me to believe I could get back in shape. When I ran cross-country in high school, I had a goal of someday running a marathon. Most marathons require a runner to be 18 to compete, so I couldn't do it in high school. I shelved the idea for the future. After law school, I moved back to New Jersey. Molly and I were engaged in October 1992. She went to work for a hospital and organized corporate wellness programs to keep people healthy. That was ironic since she was engaged to a fat and unhealthy fiancée. One program they offered to the community was called "Winners Weigh," a weight loss program through diet and exercise. Nothing new, but I participated.

I got serious about running and lost weight. My fitness improved. I remembered my goal of one day running a marathon. I tried to sign up for the 1994 New York City Marathon, but I was too late. My search for another marathon to run led me to Warwick, a small, mountainous, country town just over the New York border. I registered for that one instead.

I trained throughout the summer and into the Fall. We got married in October 1994 and went on our honeymoon in California. We got home about three weeks before the race. I made the rookie mistake of buying a new pair of sneakers in California, just weeks before the race. I didn't like them, and I had worn out my old pair, so on race day, I ran in a pair of Molly's old painting sneakers. Extremely dumb. But that was only my first mistake. There were less than 100 people in the race. I knew we would spread out over the miles, and I wanted to run with other people. I started too fast in my effort to run with others. That's devastating over a 26-mile run. The course snaked up and down around the mountains. It was a brutal day. I finished the race but had to walk much of it. I finished 40 minutes behind my goal time of 4 hours, but at least I finished! After the race, I retired from marathoning for the first time. I loved the sense of accomplishment, but I hated every step of the race.

From 1994 to 2005, I ran 11 other marathons (9 NYC marathons and 2 Philadelphia marathons), and "retired" after each one. Runners are gluttons for punishment. Since 2005, I continued running sporadically, but age, injuries, and lack of motivation plagued me. I didn't have the desire and commitment necessary to run another marathon. After several years of off and on running, I decided to train for a half-marathon. In early 2019, I was training better than I had in years. I ran three half-marathons in my fifties that were faster than any I had run in my thirties. I was ready to register for my thirteenth marathon. Unfortunately, I developed plantar fasciitis, a very painful swelling of the tendon that stretches from the Achilles heel to the toes. For almost a year, I could barely walk, let alone run. I tried injections, therapy, shoe inserts, rest, and anything my doctors could think of to get relief, but nothing worked. I got out of shape again.

Finally, I tried custom orthotics, very expensive Hoka running shoes, and Hoka slides for when I wasn't running. Over time, the pain subsided. I had my life back, and resumed running again in 2020, the year of the pandemic. What else was there to do with the entire world quarantining? My fitness improved, and I began training for another half-marathon. After completing two in early 2021, I registered for another marathon in March. It had been 16 years since my last marathon. I was nervous, but I thought I could finish it. It was not my best day, but I finished! Since then, I've run about 15 other half marathons, and completed 3 marathons in 2022.

I've had a love/hate relationship with running over the years. I used to say I'm not a runner, I'm just a person who runs. Now I realize that's not true. I am a runner. I am compelled to run, even if sometimes I don't want to. Running is part of who I am and part of who I will be for as long as I am healthy enough do to it. I used to say, "I hate running, but I do it anyway." Now I say, "I love running, the good, the bad and the ugly." I've become an addict. Running makes me feel young, healthy, fit, and whole. The good outweighs the bad and the ugly. Even after a bad run, I still have the joy of having run.

I tell you this story because there are so many parallels between the runner's life and the Christian life. I've learned many lessons about life and about our Lord Jesus Christ from running. In the Bible, there are stories of people who ran miles from one place to another to bring reports from the battlefield or to alert of approaching armies. People have been running forever. The Bible also contains figurative references to running. Paul tells us to train ourselves like runners so that we will complete the race and win the prize. The author of Hebrews tells us to run with endurance the race set before us, fixing our eyes on Jesus.

Running our race to win the prize that Jesus has set before us is every bit as grueling as running a marathon. Life is a marathon, and it's important that we train ourselves daily to run it well if we want to finish and receive the crown. Running our race for the glory of God is what this book is about. If you're a runner and you know Jesus as your Lord and Savior, you will relate to this book. I pray it encourages you on your running journey and your spiritual journey. If you don't have a relationship with God at all, or if you have allowed yourself to drift from God over the years, this book is for you, even if you're not a runner. It's time to get off the couch and get back in spiritual shape. Let's toe the starting line and get ready to run. The gun is about to go off.

CHAPTER 1

TRAINING FOR THE BIG DAY

ANY RUNNER WILL TELL you the key to running your best race is proper training and preparation. Most beginner marathon training plans schedule 18 weeks of preparation for the big day. These assume that you already have a "base." The base is the minimum fitness required to begin the training program. You should be able to run at least three miles three days a week, and six miles on the weekend before beginning the program. If you want to run a marathon, choose one that's 18 weeks away, plus however many weeks you need to build your base.

In most 18-week training programs, you'll be running 3-4 times a week, including a "long run" on the weekend, plus a day of cross training. Swimming or cycling are good cross-training options because they use different muscles. The distance of the weekday runs increases a little each week, but the long runs increase rapidly. In week 1, you'll probably run six miles. By week seven, you're up to 10 miles. By week eleven, you're running 16 miles. You'll run 20 miles in week fifteen. Then you taper. Tapering means using the final two-three weeks before the race to run less, rest more, and allow your body to recover. It's not a vacation. You'll run 12 miles two Saturdays before the race, and 8 miles the Saturday before. You should be ready for race day by week eighteen if you follow this grueling schedule. [1]

Training for a marathon takes over your life! It's not just running. You also need proper nutrition, hydration, and sleep. These are all essential to preparing to make it to the finish line. Marathon training requires massive commitment. Strict discipline is a must. Self-control is essential. While our friends are out for dinner and drinks on Friday night, runners are missing the fun. We're eating pasta and going to bed early because we want to get out early for our Saturday morning long run before it gets too hot.

Paul knew all about the discipline of training. I'm guessing that Paul never ran a marathon, although I wouldn't put it past him. Still, the same principles of strict discipline and self-control apply to our lives as Christians. Paul loved to use running as a metaphor for living out the Christian life. As a world traveler, especially in Greece, Paul likely saw many athletic competitions. They held the Isthmian Games in Greece through the first century. Paul most likely attended them. Running, boxing, wrestling and other competitions would have been among the games. Paul used some of these common activities as metaphors for how he trained his body to withstand the rigors of being a disciple of Jesus.

Paul wrote in 1 Cor. 9:24-27: "Do you not know that those who run in a race all run, but only one receives the prize? Run in such a way that you may win. Everyone who competes in the games exercises self-control in all things. So they do it to obtain a perishable wreath, but we an imperishable. Therefore I run in such a way as not to run aimlessly; I box in such a way, as to avoid hitting air; but I strictly discipline my body and make it my slave, so that, after I have preached to others, I myself will not be disqualified."

Paul was a master of metaphor. Sometimes he combined several of them in just a few verses. In this passage, Paul mentioned two athletic events, running and boxing, and the metaphor of making his body his slave. His first century readers would have understood his illustrations. Paul wasn't talking about training for a literal race or fight. He equated the Christian walk with a race or a fight; one that required strict discipline and self-control to achieve success.

He was talking about living his Christian life for the glory of God. Paul saw discipline and self-control as the keys to his life of service to Jesus. Paul never stopped training, though his training was spiritual. When we schedule a race, we know the date, so we can backfill our training schedule to be ready for race day. The only finish line a disciple of Jesus Christ ever crosses is the line from life to death to life again. Until we die, every day is race day. Of course we need time to rest, but a Christian disciple must always be prepared to work for the Lord. Every day is a day we must have trained to face. That's why Paul said to train not only to be prepared to run the race, but to win it. Paul was not content to cross the finish line. He trained to win.

Paul compared the prizes the athletes received. The winning runner received the prize, often a wreath. The winners of the Isthmian games received a crown of dried celery (yuck!) In Roman times, they changed the wreath from celery to pine. Cash prizes were also part of the victor's spoils.[2] A wreath is nice, and so is cash. But wreaths eventually fall apart, and cash gets spent. Paul talked about training to win an imperishable wreath. He meant the eternal crown that God will give us when He allows us into heaven, and Jesus says, "Well done good and faithful servant." That crown can never wear out or perish because it's given by Jesus. It will last forever. It's certainly way more valuable than a crown of celery!

This is the reason that Paul trained his body so hard. He wanted the imperishable crown that only Christ can give. That's why Paul made his body his slave. The mind controls the body, not vice versa. I have run many races in my life. I have had to walk in some of them, but I have never started a race I didn't finish. Most runners are hard-headed like me; You'd have to kill us to make us quit during a race after all that training! Paul trained his body under the discipline and self-control of his mind.

Paul used the metaphor of the flesh many times in his letters. The flesh is weak, he often said. The flesh is sinful, demanding, only seeking to satisfy its base desires. But a mind that is disciplined and self-controlled will control the body, rather than the body controlling our minds. Paul would never allow himself to lose mental and spiritual fitness, so that he would endure the grind that is Christian discipleship.

One thing I've learned in my running and racing is to respect the distance. We don't just show up on race day, not having properly trained, and think we'll be able to finish. Studies show that if we stop training even for a few weeks, we'll lose much of the fitness we've gained.[3] In the introduction, I said I "retired" from running after every marathon. I've retired more times than Brett Favre, Tom Brady and Mohammad Ali combined! My retirements never lasted long, but long enough for me to gain weight and lose fitness. Each time I unretired from marathoning, I had to start almost from zero.

Paul never retired. He never stopped training his mind, spirit, and body, so he never got out of shape. He had a plan to travel the known world planting churches in influential cities. That's exhausting work. Paul trained by praying to the Lord, studying the scriptures, and making tents to sustain himself. He built churches, strengthened the saints, and evangelized the lost. He accomplished more in his life than anyone else has for Christ because he had trained himself for the long haul. The race is long, brothers and sisters. There are few days off. Christian disciples must learn the principles of strict discipline and self-control Paul talked about in 1 Corinthians 9 to be ready to race every day.

CHAPTER 2

NEGATIVE SPLITS

A NEGATIVE SPLIT means running the second half of the race faster than the first half. I've always thought there are two ways to look at negative splits. One way is, well, negative. You didn't push hard enough in the first half and had too much energy left at the end of the race. If you ran the first half of a 10k in 33 minutes and the second half in 27 minutes, that's a bad negative split. There's too much difference between the first and second half. By spending a little more energy in the first half, you might have finished the race in 58 minutes rather than an hour.

Negative splits are positive when the second half of race is only slightly faster than the first half. That means that you've properly paced yourself and spread your energy evenly over the course of the race. You probably had enough energy left to kick it in over the last quarter mile or so, which accounts for a slightly negative split. The goal is to spend the last of your strength as you cross the finish line. It's all about learning pace, knowing your body, blocking pain, calculating endurance, and knowing when to kick it into gear to finish strong.

The opposite of a negative split is a positive split, sometimes called a positive "splat." This is when you run the first
half of the race much faster than the second. Experienced
runners sometimes plan positive splits for particular fitness
goals, but negative "splats" are typically unplanned. They
happen if we start too fast in the first half, overestimate our
stamina, then crash and burn in the second half. Maybe we
completed the race, but even if we did, it was ugly. That is a
negative "splat"!

Let's apply the positive and negative split to life. In America, most people work like dogs in their younger years, trying to
accumulate enough money so they can retire at 65 or even
younger. Once retired, many people pass their time gardening,
playing golf, watching TV, and hoping their money doesn't run
out. There's nothing wrong with those hobbies, but I think that
model is the equivalent of a positive split. We work too hard in
the early years, and by the time we get to 65, we just want to
coast in retirement. We don't have the energy or desire to finish
strong.

When I was younger and working as a lawyer, a comfortable retirement was my goal. Just the thought of twenty to
thirty more years of doing work that I didn't like caused me
tremendous stress. I didn't know what I would do with my time
once I retired, but it would be better than working as a lawyer.
They say a bad day on the golf course is better than a good day
at work. And I agree! My goals changed once I left my law
practice, started seminary, and became a pastor. I'm not yet at
retirement age, but I think little about retiring anymore. A
Christian's work is never done, and I have too much work to do!

I have a good friend who's also a pastor. His father died
recently. What a godly man he was! He planned to retire from
his career as an architect at 60, not to play golf, but to work as a
missionary. He enjoyed a successful 30-year career, but all the

while, he was saving so he could spend the last years of his life in full-time service to the Lord. After he "retired," he used the money he had saved to travel overseas, lending his skills to help design and build churches and schools for disadvantaged kids. He spread the gospel wherever he went. Now that's a retirement plan!

When I was working as a lawyer and considering the rest of my life, I read a book by Bob Buford, called *Halftime*. Buford encouraged people to consider how they want to spend the second half of their lives and plan accordingly. Halftime is a purposeful time of reflection to catch a new vision for the second half of your life. Buford wrote, "My passion is to multiply all that God has given me, and in the process, give it back."[1] That book helped motivate me to leave my law career and pursue ministry in my forties. This architect turned missionary did the same. His second half of life was even more productive than his first.

Unfortunately, he got cancer when he turned about 80. As he lay dying, he encouraged the nurses who ministered to him. When he couldn't talk anymore, he could still smile. And that's what he did, right to the end. At his memorial service, so many people he ministered to after he retired spoke lovingly of him. His impact post-retirement will echo throughout the generations.

His life race was a negative split. For the glory of God, He ran the second half of his life faster than the first. He understood the right way to pace his life, working, providing for his family in the first half, and saving for the second half. After he retired from his career, he gave almost twenty years of his life to ministry. He sprinted through the finish line, smiling the whole time. When he died, he heard the glorious words that the Lord Jesus spoke to him, "Well done, good and faithful servant."

. . .

I want Jesus to speak those words to me. I don't want to waste the last years of my life that I could spend serving Him. Golf is great and taking a day or two to relax is fine, but I want to run a negative split. If my health holds up and the Lord wills, that's what I plan to do. Many people in their golden years think they have nothing to offer, or they're too tired to serve others. I believe that if we have breath in our lungs, God can use us. We each have God-given talents, experience, and wisdom. God gave us these gifts to minister to others. They don't expire when we turn 65. We can use them until the day we die if we are willing. Don't slow down. Finish strong and run a negative split.

CHAPTER 3

BELONGING

I RAN in a race called the "Too Hot to Handle" half-marathon in Dallas last summer. The "swag," (that's the stuff they give you for entering the race) for the THTH included a red sport tech tank top with white piping around the shoulders and neck. It's my favorite summer running tank, so I wear it often. I was wearing it the other day as I was running one of my usual trails. As I did, I passed a lady about my age, maybe a little younger, wearing the same race shirt. She said, "nice shirt." I had to look down to remember what shirt I was wearing, but I recovered quickly. I said, "I like yours too." We shared a smile and continued in opposite directions. It was maybe a two second encounter, but it made me feel good.

It's a fact of life that it will be hot in Texas in July. The THTH race day was a scorcher. I had just gotten over a cold, and the heat and humidity didn't help. I had to walk parts of it and stumbled over the finish line well over my regular pace. This lady who was a stranger to me experienced the same heat on the same course that I did. I don't know how she performed, but she probably wouldn't wear the shirt if she didn't finish.

(Most runners adhere to the unwritten rule that says you don't wear the shirt if you didn't finish the race.) I may never see her again. I would only recognize her if I saw her in the same shirt at the same place. Even so, we had a shared experience. We belonged not only to a community of runners, but to an even smaller community of people who ran the same race in that awful heat.

We all want to belong to something. The human heart craves community. That's why family and friends are so important to us. We need our people. Running is usually the opposite of community living. We spend hours and hours alone running the same trails, lost in our thoughts, pacing ourselves, counting down the miles and minutes until we're done. My encounter with that woman made me remember that even though I run alone, I'm part of something much larger. I belong to a community of runners who share my passion. We're a small community, but these are my people, even though we've never met. They understand me in a way that non-runners don't. We have mutual shared experiences. All long-time runners know the injuries, boredom, suffering, and lack of motivation on the one hand, but the thrill of finishing a race, or setting a personal record, or just the joy of completing a run on the other. The runner's life is full of highs and lows, and we runners have a special bond with each other because we experience them all.

That same principle now applies to belonging to a church. When I was young, I never wanted to go to church on Sunday. It was so long, so boring, and so early! Now that I'm a believer and pastor of a church, I love going to church on Sunday. I spend about half my time alone, reading, researching, and preparing my sermon for Sunday. The church I pastor has about 100 members and most Sundays, about 70 people attend. These are my people, my community. We share a bond of faith in Jesus Christ and the knowledge that we will all spend eternity in heaven together.

The first century church shared this same bond. Christianity was brand new in Acts 2. Jesus had recently risen from the dead and ascended into heaven. Before He went, He told his apostles to go to Jerusalem and wait to receive the Holy Spirit. The Holy Spirit came at Pentecost and indwelt the new believers. They became part of God's new creation called the church. Acts 2:42-47 recounts how they lived in community together.

"They were continually devoting themselves to the apostles' teaching and to fellowship, to the breaking of bread and to prayer. Everyone kept feeling a sense of awe; and many wonders and signs were taking place through the apostles. And all those who had believed were together and had all things in common; and they *began* selling their property and possessions and were sharing them with all, as anyone might have need. Day by day continuing with one mind in the temple, and breaking bread from house to house, they were taking their meals together with gladness and sincerity of heart, praising God and having favor with all the people. And the Lord was adding to their number day by day those who were being saved."

Like love of running joins runners, these people became a community bonded only by love for Jesus. In America, we don't enjoy community fellowship like the first century church. We "schedule" community events, and have our occasional potluck dinners, but in first century Israel, they lived life in community. They understood its value.

The reason I love race day so much is that I finally get to be with like-minded people. I'm not that chatty on race morning, but there's something comforting about being with a group of people who understand each other. We run the same race together. Don't get me wrong, I'm competitive by nature! I want to do my best and if I could beat every runner out there, I would. But I am also a realist and know that I'm not winning any races. The genuine joy is in sharing the experience together and listening to the stories when the race is over. That's the same reason I love being in church, running the race of life together and sharing stories of how Jesus has poured His grace into our lives. Cherish your encounters with other Christians, as I cherished my brief encounter with the woman wearing the same shirt. We belong to a small community bonded by God's love and grace.

CHAPTER 4

DISCIPLINE

ELIUD KIPCHOGE of Kenya won the gold medal in the men's marathon at the 2020 Tokyo Olympics (which were held in 2021 because of the Covid epidemic). The temperature hovered in the upper 80s with high humidity. Kipchoge dominated the field, cruising to the finish line, and smiling over the last 10k. I watched him tearing up the streets of Tokyo in disbelief. His average pace per mile was about 4:50! I researched his training regimen. He runs every day, and twice a day several days a week. His *short* runs are 16-21km, which equates to about 10-13 miles. He incorporates sprint work on the track with interval training, short runs, and long runs, logging well over 100 miles a week. Obviously, running is his full-time job, so he has the time. But can you imagine the discipline required to keep that schedule? When does he rest?!

My motivation to maintain physical fitness waxes and wanes. For several months, I might dedicate myself to training and losing weight. After a while, and especially when I've just completed a marathon, I grow tired and my desire fades. It feels like reaching the mountaintop, and then there's nothing left to do. So, I allow myself some time off, lose my self-discipline, gain a few pounds, and get out of shape. I've always tried to avoid this cycle, but as I said in the introduction, I've retired after every marathon. It takes prolonged discipline to stay physically fit enough to spend your life running. My strategy to defeat the post-marathon malaise is to sign up for another marathon. But man, I get tired.

Now that I'm in my mid-fifties, it gets harder each day to get out the door to run. Aches and pains are more common. Morning stiffness is real. When I was a boy, I'd hop out of bed and hit the ground running. As a young father, I always knew when our son Brian was awake. He would break the silence of the morning with his feet. We would hear nothing, and then, bam, bam, bam, bam, bam, as his feet hit the floor. Like me at his age, he was running wherever he went. As we age, it gets harder to get moving, and especially to lace up our shoes for a run. We must force our bodies to do what they don't want to do to reach our fitness goals.

Our walk with God is much the same way. Paul wrote in Romans 12:1-2: "Therefore, I urge you, brethren, by the mercies of God, to present your bodies a living and holy sacrifice, acceptable to God, which is your spiritual service of worship." We often find ourselves at the crossroads of choosing between what we want and what God wants. God places us in situations to train us to live sacrificially and to serve. We need discipline to choose to serve God rather than ourselves. I admire Kipchoge's discipline. But the discipline required to offer ourselves as living sacrifices is even greater. It requires supernatural self-control that only the Holy Spirit can give. First century Jews offered animal sacrifices to atone for their sins. They burned up the entire animal. That's what Paul meant about offering our bodies as living sacrifices. We don't die physically as the animals did, but we offer all of ourselves up for service. We can only do this by obeying the Holy Spirit rather than our own desires. (I've heard, and it always stayed with me, that the trouble with living sacrifices is that they keep crawling off the altar!) It's a decision to stay there and offer ourselves as a sacrifice.

Galatians 5:17 says: "For the flesh sets its desire against the Spirit, and the Spirit against the flesh; for these are in opposition to one another." A constant battle rages between our human desires, which Paul calls "the flesh," and the will of the Holy Spirit. The Holy Spirit empowers us to fight against our flesh, to live a life of sacrifice and service to each other. We naturally resist that lifestyle because we are by nature selfish creatures. We want to do what makes us happy and comfortable. When God calls us to sacrifice or service, our flesh says, "Relax. Someone else will handle it." That's not what God wants. Christians have the Holy Spirit who lives in us, training us to live a sacrificial life of service. When we see a person in need, the Holy Spirit works in us, and we can't turn away. He compels us to help even if we might prefer to do something else. We don't develop this discipline overnight. It takes years of habit building.

Runners understand this ongoing battle. Every morning we face the temptation to blow off the morning run and spend another hour in bed. It's too cold, too hot, too wet, too early. We're too tired, too sore, or too lazy. In that moment, our trained minds decide to hit the road over the objection of our bodies. We put our feet in our sneakers and head out the door. If you're not a runner, think about it like going to work. Each morning you may wake up with ten reasons to call in sick. It's a learned discipline to get in the shower, get dressed, and get yourself to work.

Success in any part of life requires discipline. Students must go to class and study to earn good grades. Employees work hard to climb the corporate ladder. Pastors spend lonely hours preparing messages to feed and shepherd their flock. Runners train their brains to tell their bodies it's time to run. The body objects, but the mind controls the body. The discipline of running comes from deep within.

Sacrifice and service are disciplines as well. When we have the choice of service or comfort, what will we do? Will we find an escape hatch that will allow us to ride the couch, or will we deny our flesh to serve God? As we train ourselves to serve God, we'll stop looking for escape hatches. Instead, we'll increasingly ignore our flesh and volunteer to do what needs to be done. If you've run for a long time, you understand. Your body doesn't even bother to object anymore. It's going for a run, even though it doesn't want to.

Your body becomes the slave of whatever your mind wills. The more we run, the more we'll enjoy running. It becomes part of who we are. We can do the same in service to others. Don't get me wrong, rest is crucial for the body. Too much rest becomes laziness though, so balance is the key. Through supernatural discipline that the Holy Spirit will develop in us, we can serve God even when we'd prefer not to. Over time, the voice of the flesh grows quiet as the power of the Holy Spirit leads us to serve.

CHAPTER 5

COMPARISON

A RACE IS A COMPETITION. The nature of competition is to compare ourselves with others to see who is the fastest. The fastest runner wins the race. By comparison, the rest of the runners are slower. I haven't won a race since high school. But I don't race to compare myself to others. At my age, I'd leave every race feeling like a failure. I couldn't beat the twenty-somethings when I was twenty-something.

In most races, runners can win awards by their age bracket. When I was 54, I was the oldest in the 50-54 age bracket. I never won my age category. In 2021, I was 55, among the youngest in the 55-59 age bracket. That year, I won my age bracket in a local 5k. OK, so there were only 5 people in my age bracket, but still! It was a race, and I won! I placed 11th out of 120 in my age bracket in one half marathon this year, and 9th out of 28 in another. Some races even award trophies for placing in the top three of each age group. Who knew?! I admit I enjoy winning awards. But I don't want to get in the habit of comparing myself to other runners. My finishing position has more to do with who else entered the race than with me. If you lined up the fifty fastest 55–59-year-olds in Texas, I'd come in last. If you lined up the slowest, I'd finish first. All I can do is run my race. If I'm pleased with my time, I try not to care where I finished. (I still do care. But I try not to.) Comparison will only lead to pride if I finish close to the top, or shame and embarrassment if I finish close to the bottom.

Comparison is dangerous in our walk with the Lord too. It's human nature to compare ourselves with others, even in our spiritual lives. Comparing our spiritual lives will always result in pride or shame. Take the super-spiritual Christian who reads his Bible an hour a day, prays an hour a day, and does some act of service every day. Let's call him, "pious man." If he does those things with a pure and sincere heart, he's a strong Christian. Lord knows we need more of them. But let's say "pious man" starts comparing himself to someone who only has 10 minutes a day to read his Bible and pray because he works two jobs to feed his family. Let's call him "busy man." Comparison will make pious man proud, and pride is a sin.

Let's look at my hypothetical from busy man's perspective. If he compared himself with pious man, he might feel shame, embarrassment, remorse, and maybe even guilt that he doesn't do enough. That's taking the grace that Jesus died for and saying, "It isn't enough, I also must work hard." I've heard the quote "comparison is the thief of joy" and I believe it! The danger of comparison is when we compare down, we feel badly about ourselves. When we compare up, we become proud and judgmental. Jesus showed the danger of comparison in the parable He told in Luke 18:9-14:

> "And He also told this parable to some people who
> trusted in themselves that they were righteous, and
> viewed others with contempt: Two men went up into
> the temple to pray, one a Pharisee and the other a tax

collector. The Pharisee stood and was praying this to himself: 'God, I thank You that I am not like other people: swindlers, unjust, adulterers, or even like this tax collector. I fast twice a week; I pay tithes of all that I get.' But the tax collector, standing some distance away, was even unwilling to lift up his eyes to heaven, but was beating his breast, saying, 'God, be merciful to me, the sinner!' I tell you, this man went to his house justified rather than the other; for everyone who exalts himself will be humbled, but he who humbles himself will be exalted."

The Pharisee compared himself with the tax collector and deemed himself worthy of God's blessing. His problem was that he thought he was righteous because of the good deeds he did. He trusted in himself and his good deeds to enter the kingdom of heaven. He misunderstood the standard required to get into heaven. It's not by setting an arbitrary standard and then meeting it. The standard to get into heaven is perfection. Since we all sin, none of us is perfect. We all need a savior, no matter how highly we think of ourselves. That's the danger of comparing ourselves to others instead of judging ourselves by God's holy standard.

If pious man compares himself to busy man, rather than acknowledging that he's desperately in need of a savior, he'll become like the Pharisee in this parable. His Bible reading, prayer, and service will become a source of pride that will keep him out of heaven. He won't have the humility required to admit that he's a sinner in need of a savior. That's why Jesus warned against comparison.

On the flip side, the tax collector compared himself with God's standard of perfection and knew he fell short. God blessed the tax collector because of his humility. If busy man compares himself to God's standard and understands that salvation is of the Lord and not of his works, he won't feel ashamed that he can't keep pious man's standards. He knows Jesus died for his sins. He's placed his faith in Jesus for salvation, and he measures his spiritual growth not in *minutes* spent reading the Bible, but in a *life* spent in service to the Lord.

When you toe the line at a race, it's ok to want to beat the guy next to you. But our spiritual walk is not a competition, nor should we compare ourselves to others. God has given us each our own race to run. We should strive to love Jesus the best we can without comparing ourselves to others. We'll never know "pious man's" heart. Only Jesus knows that. He knows your heart too. Run your spiritual race as well as you can, giving God the glory, and don't worry about how you stack up against others. There is no first place or last place when we cross the finish line of our spiritual race. There's only Jesus, who says to us, "Well done, good and faithful slave. You were faithful with a few things, I will put you in charge of many things; enter the joy of your master" (Matthew 25:21.)

CHAPTER 6

INTROVERTED

RUNNING suits my personality because I do it alone. It's not that I'm shy. I like people! But if I could choose between attending a big party full of strangers, or reading in my office, I'm reading in my office every time. You might say I'm an introvert, and you'd be right!

An introvert is "a person who prefers calm environments, limits social engagement, or embraces a greater than average preference for solitude."[1] That describes me well. I've taken the Meyers-Briggs personality test several times. Each time, the results tell me I am an ISTJ. The "I" stands for introverted. I'm a very strong "I." I spend a lot of time alone at my desk, writing sermons, blog posts, or working on a book. When I'm not, I'm either out running or walking, or home with my wife. I like to go out and have fun. Concerts, baseball games, races, and festivals, are some of my favorite things, but I prefer to be anonymous in a crowd. Extroverts draw energy from large crowds, whereas introverts spend energy in social situations. Introverts need to recharge after social situations by spending time alone.[2]

. . .

I can't prove it, but my gut tells me that Jesus was an introvert too. Jesus loved people. He wanted them to come to Him and receive salvation. But people always wanted something from Him. Some wanted healing. Others wanted to test Him and trap Him in His words. Either way, people exhausted Jesus. After He spoke to the masses, He needed to be alone to recharge His batteries and to pray. He spent hours and even nights with God the Father on the mountains and hills of Israel, praying and recharging for the day ahead.

In Matthew 14 for example, Jesus received the news that Herod murdered John the Baptist. Matthew 14:13 says: "Now when Jesus heard about John, He withdrew from there in a boat to a secluded place by Himself." But the people watched His boat and ran around the small lake they called the Sea of Galilee to meet him. Matthew 14:14 says: "When He came ashore, He saw a large crowd, and felt compassion for them and healed their sick." When it became late and the people had no food, he took five loaves and two fish that a young boy had brought and fed over 5000 people with them. After that long day, he sent his disciples away on a boat to the other side of the lake while he dispersed the crowds. Matthew 14:23: "After He had sent the crowds away, He went up on the mountain by Himself to pray; and when it was evening, He was there alone." Not much later, a storm arose. Jesus came to His disciples walking on the water, calmed them and the sea. They came to land, the people recognized Him, and He began healing again.

Throughout the gospels, we see the cycle that He was among the people, and then went off to be alone in prayer. I understand. People can drain us if we don't set boundaries. Even Jesus established boundaries to give Himself time with His Father to recharge. One appeal of running is the time I spend alone. When I started running years ago, I carried a Sony Walkman and listened to cassette tapes! (Kids, ask your parents!) In the thirty years or so that I've been running as an adult, the technology has improved. Now I wear a Garmin watch and listen to music or podcasts through my airpods.

Running allows me another hour of solitude before I begin my workday. I often use that time to listen to sermons from preachers I enjoy. Some of my closest friends are pastors, and I love to spend time with them in the word as they preach. As I listen to them, I learn so much about God, but also about the art of preaching. Preachers' methods and styles differ, but the word of God never changes. Listening to them challenges me to be a better preacher and helps me understand the passage they are preaching better.

Since starting a new journey as an author, I now listen to podcasts about self-publishing too. Self-publishing was a mystery to me when I started my first book. Listening to podcasts while running has taught me so much. I pray I will write many more books and that each one brings glory to God. It's clear to me that God has brought my desire to run and my introverted nature together to bring glory to Himself. I've used the time I spend alone on the roads to learn about God; to inspire ideas for writing; and to learn how to put pen to paper and turn those ideas into blogs, sermons, and books.

I have often wished that I was extroverted. People who can walk into a party and feel completely at ease amaze me. Some people have never met a stranger. I would love to have that quality. But the world needs introverts too. We can't all be the life of the party. Jesus could only stand to be the center of attention for a little at a time, then He withdrew to be with His Father. If you're an introvert like me, you're in good company! Use the time alone to recharge your batteries, learn more about God, and how He might want to use you for His kingdom.

CHAPTER 7

A BOND EVEN STRONGER
THAN FAMILY

I USUALLY SEE at least a dozen other runners on my morning runs. Runners are creatures of habit. We run the same trails because we know our mile markers. We know how far we've come and how far until we're home. I don't know any of the local runners, but since we see each other frequently, we give each other a warm smile and wave. It's not a high five, but it's more than a perfunctory nod too. We runners are a special breed. We understand each other at some level, though we may share nothing else in common, almost like an extended family.

This morning I ran in the rain. I like to get my run out of the way in the morning. If I don't, then I'll eat breakfast, start reading emails or working on my sermon, and before I know it, the day is gone. So I went out even though it was raining. It's not like I got caught in the rain. It was raining when I left the house. If passing runners on a sunny day is like seeing your extended family, meeting runners who are out in the rain is like seeing your immediate family. Who goes out running in the rain? Not casual runners. Only serious, dedicated runners do. When we pass each other on wet roads, we share a knowing smile, because we share a special kinship that's even stronger than our bond with sunny day runners. I feel united with these rainy-day runners even though we've never met.

We might expect that Jesus shared a strong bond with His family. His mother Mary received special knowledge of who He was. Surely, His brothers and sisters knew the circumstances of Jesus' birth and the prophecies from the angel Gabriel and the old priest Simeon. Some might also think Jesus shared a special bond with His own people, the scribes and Pharisees, who were also Jews. Yet, when Jesus was in the middle of His ministry, the scribes and Pharisees hated Him, and His own family thought He was crazy. Let's look at the scribes and Pharisees first. In Mark 3, Jesus entered a synagogue and met a man with a withered hand. It was the Sabbath, and according to the traditions of the Pharisees, it was against the law of Moses to work on the Sabbath. The Pharisees were waiting for Jesus to heal the man so they would have something against Him. Jesus healed the man. Instead of being amazed and praising God, His actions outraged the Pharisees. They went out to plot how they might kill Him!

So, Jesus left there and went to the sea of Galilee to choose His disciples. He chose Judas, knowing he would betray Him, but chose none from His family. Why would He do that? At this point in His ministry, even Judas hoped Jesus was the promised Messiah. His own brothers didn't. After, Jesus returned home to Galilee, and such a large crowd gathered that He couldn't even eat, but none of His brothers or sisters were present. The people started arguing about Jesus. The scribes said Jesus cast out demons by the ruler of the demons, meaning Satan. Jesus replied, "How can Satan cast out Satan? A house divided against itself cannot stand."

What about His family? He shared the same mother with His brothers and sisters, but when they heard He was back in town, "they went out to take custody of Him; for they were saying, 'He has lost his senses'" (Mark 3:21). When His mother and brothers arrived, those crowded inside the house let Him know they were there. They said, "Behold, Your mother and Your brothers are outside looking for You." Answering them, He said, "Who are My mother and My brothers?" Looking about at those who were sitting around Him, He said, "Behold My mother and My brothers! For whoever does the will of God, he is My brother and sister and mother" (Mark 3:32-35.)

Blood is thicker than water, but faith is thicker than blood. In other words, it's shared faith rather than blood that makes us part of the family of God. I imagine those who heard Jesus' statement felt a special kinship with Jesus. His fellow Jews and His own family shared blood, ethnicity, or heritage, but Jesus said His true family were those who did the will of God. In John 6:40, Jesus said, "For this is the will of My Father, that everyone who beholds the Son and believes in Him will have eternal life, and I Myself will raise him up on the last day." Those gathered with Jesus, who believed in Him though they did not share family blood, were His genuine family.

Most of us love our earthly families dearly, even though some may be unbelievers. We share the gospel with them hoping that one day they will believe, and that they will spend eternity in heaven too. But we will spend eternity with our spiritual family. When we go to church on Sunday, we worship the Lord with our congregation. We also know there are millions of people in churches around the world worshiping our Savior too! We'll never meet most of these believers, but we share a deep bond. These are our spiritual family.

Runners come from different ethnicities and heritage, but we share this common love of running. We don't stop and talk to each other during runs because we're too dialed into our run. We're busy checking our watches, thinking about our pace and breathing, monitoring aches and pains, and budgeting oxygen and energy for the balance of the run. But that's ok. The bond still runs deep. I feel an even deeper connection to other rainy-day runners. We're intense, driven, and determined to achieve our goals. I don't know if these runners are part of my eternal family. Only God knows that. I'm a member of a Facebook Group called "Christian Runners." Its mission statement is: "Utilizing God's gift of running to further His Kingdom through fellowship, community, and service." I only know these runners from chatting with them over Facebook, but what a joy it is to know that we share, not only the love of running, but the love of Christ! That's an unbreakable bond.

CHAPTER 8

ENCOURAGEMENT

I HAVE STARTED and completed nine New York City Marathons. I can tell you it's a lot easier to start than to finish. The race begins on the Verrazano-Narrows Bridge in Staten Island. The bridge crosses from Staten Island to Brooklyn. At about the halfway point in the race, runners cross from Brooklyn into Queens. The 59th Street bridge carries runners from Queens to Manhattan at the 16-mile mark. That's a hard part of the race because the bridge inclines sharply for about a mile before descending for a mile, and there are no spectators on the bridge to cheer you on. A lot of runners start walking at this point of the race. Coming off the bridge, huge crowds at least 10 people deep greet the runners, who then proceed about four miles north on First Avenue before crossing the Willis Avenue Bridge into the Bronx near the 20-mile mark. Only about a mile of the course is in the Bronx. Runners return to Manhattan via the Madison Avenue Bridge. They continue south on 5th Avenue into Central Park, running around the southern end of Central Park before crossing the finish line.

· · ·

If I remember correctly, the story I'm about to tell you happened during the 1995 New York City Marathon. I had crossed the Willis Avenue Bridge into the Bronx. Twenty miles into the race and I felt it. I was moving so slowly that I had lost contact with other runners in front of me and behind me. There I was all alone, practically crawling through the Bronx, when an African American spectator said to me, "Son, you're in the Bronx now. You better start runnin' a whole lot faster than that!" I wasn't sure if he was threatening, warning, or encouraging me! Anyway, his words added a little pep to my step for a while. Sometimes you just need proper motivation!

Runners love encouragement. Spectators cheering and carrying signs motivate us to run well. My favorite sign is from a female spectator I've seen at a few races that says, "You have stamina. Call me!" That makes me laugh and gives me a little shot of energy to carry me a little further. Racing can be discouraging, especially if we've trained hard and long and we're just not having our best day. We need the encouragement from others to supply what is lacking in our own strength and stamina.

Our Christian walk is similar. Life and discouragement seem to go hand in hand. Whether you watch the news on TV or read it on Google, you're bound to be discouraged. If you're a Christian watching the world abandon God and His morals and values, it's very disheartening. So where can a Christian find encouragement in the world? My first source is the Bible. It's chock full of verses God put in there so when we're tempted to quit, we'll remember that He loves us and He's in control. I would like to see some of these Bible verses on signs as I run.

Psalm 27:12: "The LORD is my light and my salvation; whom shall I fear? The LORD is the stronghold of my life; of whom shall I be afraid?" Romans 8:31: "If God is for us, who can be against us?" Isaiah 41:10: "Fear not, for I am with you; be not dismayed, for I am your God; I will strengthen you, I will help you, I will uphold you with my righteous right hand." Philippians 4:13: "I can do all things through him who strengthens me." I could fill a book with the Bible's encouraging verses. In fact, God already has. That's why we ought to read it!

One of the Bible's best encouragers was Barnabas. Barnabas was full of the Holy Spirit and faith. Some people are "cross the street" people. When you see them coming, you cross the street. Barnabas wasn't one of them. No one was ever unhappy about running into Barnabas. He was the kind of guy that would always make you feel better about yourself. Don't you want to be a Barnabas? I know how to encourage others, even though I'm not always good at doing it. Smile a lot. Genuinely care about other people. Listen. Seek people out and encourage them. Tell them that God loves them and that His plan and timing for them is perfect. Just be a friend to people. Barnabas attracted people and because of that, he won many to Christ.

My wife is my great encourager. She's my biggest supporter. She's always in my corner. When life is hard, she holds me up and points me back to Jesus. God calls all Christians to lift each other up. In 1 Thessalonians 5, Paul exhorted the Christians in the church to build each other up. He reminded them that the Lord could come at any moment in judgment, but Christians do not need to fear. He wrote, "For God has not destined us for wrath, but for obtaining salvation through our Lord Jesus Christ, who died for us, so that whether we are awake or asleep, we will live together with Him. Therefore encourage one another and build up one another, just as you also are doing" (1 Thessalonians 5:9-11).

I love those verses. Whenever I preside over a funeral, I always include them. Life is hard. Death waits at the end of it unless Jesus returns first. But Christians should not fear. Paul encouraged his readers that God has not planned wrath for believers, but salvation! Sometimes the Christian life can be a lot like running a marathon. It's easier to start it than to finish it. We need to encourage others to complete the race using verses like this from the Bible. There's no better reassurance than God's word spoken to us by another believer. When I was running through the Bronx, it wasn't God's word, but fear that kept me running! God's word is so much better than fear. It gives us hope, which in the Bible means the certainty that God will deliver all He has promised. Take heart, believer. Be encouraged. God will get you across the finish line.

CHAPTER 9

RUNNING BEFORE SUNRISE

SUMMERS IN TEXAS ARE HOT! From mid-June to mid-September, the mercury rises to near 100 degrees every day. If I want to get my run in, it's got to be early. By 8 a.m., it's too hot for me. That means I often get up at 5:30, hoping to be on the road by 6. By late August, as the days are getting shorter again, it's still pitch dark at 6 a.m.

One early morning on the road, I noticed the darkness giving way to light every minute. By 6:30, the sky was bright. I love watching the night sky transition to daylight. When I left the house, the moon glowed. I saw hundreds of stars. The change happened almost imperceptibly. Second by second, the sun's light swallowed up the stars I could see so clearly only minutes ago. Birds, squirrels, and rabbits hidden by the darkness became visible. Light reveals what the darkness hides. In just a few minutes' time, light chased the darkness away.

John 8:12 says: "Then Jesus again spoke to them, saying, 'I am the Light of the world; the one who follows Me will not walk in the darkness, but will have the Light of life.'" Salvation is like the dawn of a new day. Once we walked in spiritual darkness, not knowing the depth of our sin or our need for a Savior. Somehow, God calls us out of the darkness and into the light of the gospel of salvation. For some, the transition happens quickly. I've heard testimonies of people who said that they were unbelievers and then, in an instant, God changed their hearts. C. S. Lewis said of his conversion:

"When we set out, I did not believe that Jesus Christ was the Son of God, but when we reached the zoo I did. I had not exactly spent the journey in thought, nor in dominant emotion. 'Emotional' is perhaps the last word we can apply to some of the most important events. It was more like when a man, after a long sleep, still lying motionless on the bed, becomes aware that he is now awake." [1]

For Lewis, God instantly lifted the darkness and filled His world with light. My journey to faith didn't happen in a flash like it does for some people. My conversion took over a year. I was a tough nut to crack! Slowly but surely, just as night becomes day, God showed me the truth of His Word and the beauty of His Son. He called me to himself by putting people and resources in my life to convince me of the truth of the gospel. Some of those circumstances were incredibly painful. But God had to till the hard earth of my heart before He could plant the seeds of faith that would bloom.

When we hear about people who seem to be "overnight successes," it may seem that way from our perspective. Likely, the foundation of their success was many years of work and preparation that we weren't present to see. I think the same is true when we hear about instantaneous conversions to Christianity. It may seem instantaneous to the new believer. However, before God can save, He must draw that person to Himself by His Holy Spirit and through some of life's difficult circumstances. This takes time. Slowly, God causes the darkness to fade as He fills our hearts with light. We can measure the transition from night to day in minutes and seconds. God's work in lifting the spiritual darkness may take years. Everyone who has experienced God's love has a different testimony. The essentials are the same. God caused us to see the depth of our sin and our need for a savior. The difference is in the details. We all will have a unique story of how God chased the darkness and filled our lives with light. He can do that with our unbelieving family and friends too. Is anyone beyond God's reach? If I wasn't, then no one is.

On these early mornings, when I get dressed and get ready to run, I gaze at the blackness out my window and wonder how long I'll be running before I have enough light to see. I never wonder *if* the light will come; it always *does*. I glorify God for a new day. As the sun creeps over the horizon, it reminds me that God revealed His light to me when I was in darkness. If He would do that for me, why wouldn't He do it for family and friends who have not yet received Jesus as Savior? I pray they will no longer walk in darkness but will have the Light of life. For all you early morning runners, as the night becomes day, think about how God lifted the spiritual darkness from your heart so you would believe the gospel and become His child. Pray that He would do the same for your family and friends, and then glorify Him for His grace.

CHAPTER 10

PORTA POTTIES

I'VE RUN plenty of long races. There are so many things to think about! Nutrition, hydration, band-aids, Vaseline to prevent chafing, the proper clothing, sneakers, and after race necessities are just a few examples. Runners pack these items the night before, so we have them on race day. We also choose what we're going to wear the night prior to the race, so we're not frantically tearing through our laundry looking for our favorite shorts on race day. Runners want to eliminate all the variables we can. We don't want any surprises. Preparation is the key to a successful race. There's always one big unknown though, our bladders. The longest lines at the porta-potties form ten minutes before the race. Everyone wants to be sure they're empty before they start. God has blessed me with a pretty good bladder. I almost never have to stop during the race, even if I'm running a full marathon. But there have been a few times when I had no choice.

I hate losing my position against other runners in the race. They gain while I drain. Then there's the race against the clock. It keeps running while I'm not. I also hate losing my rhythm. I spend more energy restarting and finding my stride than I would if I hadn't stopped. But even worse than those annoyances, is the dread of opening the porta-potty door. As a mid-pack runner, by the time I need a potty break, the porta-potties are well "broken-in," shall we say. I gingerly open the door and wince as though a bomb may explode. Often, it already has. I only see the aftermath. I advance my nose forward an inch at a time, determining just how bad this might be. Finally, the moment of truth, I'm losing time, so in I go.

A porta-potty is a lot like life sometimes. You never know what you're gonna get. Sometimes it's great. Other times it really stinks, and you just hold your nose and get through it. Life is unpredictable. We never know what tomorrow will bring. Proverbs 14:27 says, "Do not boast about tomorrow, for you don't know what a day may bring." James 4:13-14 says: "Now listen, you who say, 'Today or tomorrow we will go to this or that city, spend a year there, carry on business and make money.' Why, you do not even know what will happen tomorrow. What is your life? You are a mist that appears for a little while and then vanishes."

Here's one thing we shouldn't do and one thing we should. We shouldn't waste time worrying. Jesus told the people in Matthew 6:34: "Therefore do not worry about tomorrow, for tomorrow will worry about itself. Each day has enough trouble of its own." Worry is foolish because it doesn't solve any of our problems. We don't know what's going to happen tomorrow, so why worry about it? Instead, we should put our lives in God's hands and trust God with the outcome.

What we should do is prepare. If I want to avoid the porta-potty during a race, I don't eat sausage and peppers the night before as much as I love it. I eat pasta and other carbohydrates. I don't drink a gallon of water an hour before the race. If I've hydrated well in the preceding days, I only need a little water on race morning. In life, we should prepare for two certainties: trials and eternity. Regarding trials, Jesus promised in John 16:33: "I have told you these things, so that in me you may have peace. In this world you will have trouble. But take heart! I have overcome the world." The reason Jesus told us about the trials we will face in advance is so that we might have peace. Be prepared for trials by knowing they are coming and having peace that God is in control.

Regarding eternity, Hebrews 9:27-28 says: "Just as people are destined to die once, and after that to face judgment, so Christ was sacrificed once to take away the sins of many; and He will appear a second time, not to bear sin, but to bring salvation to those who are waiting for him." We're all going to die unless Jesus returns first. Whether we die before He returns or He returns while we're still alive, we will see Him face to face. His judgment is based on whether we have trusted Him for salvation. If we have, we have nothing to fear.

Many people go through life not knowing if they are going to heaven. They are afraid to die and face it like a runner might face a porta-potty door, not knowing what's behind it, and with much fear and trembling. There's no reason for that. Prepare yourself now for Jesus' return. Proper preparation can eliminate many of life's uncertainties. We can know for sure that we're going to heaven if we've trusted Jesus for salvation.

CHAPTER 11

INJURIES

I RAN two half marathons in Spring 2019 after not having run one for about two years. I was happy to be back in shape, but toward the summer I started having severe pain in my right foot. In June 2019, I ran a race called the Hero Hustle half marathon. I shouldn't have run it, but I can be very stubborn (and stupid.) By the time I finished, I could barely walk. It felt like walking on glass. I had to go see a doctor for the pain. I had heard of plantar fasciitis but had no idea what it was. Turns out there's a tendon that extends from your heel to your toes called the plantar fascia. It can become inflamed and irritated through overuse. The doctor said I would need plenty of rest. I tried that, plus injections and physical therapy. Nothing helped. That injury sidelined me for nearly a year before someone suggested that I try orthotics and very stable running shoes. It took a while, but that combination changed my life. The pain went away, and I could walk again, and then run. As of now, I'm healthy and running.

. . .

All runners deal with injuries. We do our best to prevent them, but some are unavoidable. Accidents are a leading cause of injury. We could trip over a sidewalk crack or a curb. I once kicked a sprinkler head while walking to the starting line of a race. It was still dark and I couldn't see it. I saw stars and wasn't sure I'd be able to run. I got through it though. Other times, injuries occur from our aging bodies breaking down under the stress of running. The best way to avoid injury is to be careful and to listen to our bodies. Watch out for sprinkler heads and don't be afraid to take a day off.

Injuries are unwanted interruptions of our plans. We write out a training schedule and intend to stick to it. When the unexpected and dreaded injuries derail our schedule, we really get upset. Speaking for myself, if I lose a few days to a minor injury, I can live with it. But after a week or so, I know I'm losing fitness and I become severely agitated. I don't want my training interrupted. Jesus suffered no bodily injury until the crucifixion as far as we know. But injured people interrupted Him all the time. He never seemed to mind. It's as though He planned for interruptions and made room for them in His schedule.

One of Jesus's most famous interrupters was the woman who had been bleeding for twelve years. A man named Jairus, a synagogue official, came to ask Jesus to come heal his dying daughter. As Jesus walked with Jairus to his home, this woman came up behind Jesus and touched His cloak. She believed touching Him would heal her. Jesus felt power go out from Him, and He stopped to ask who touched Him. The woman bowed and humbly confessed. Jesus said that her faith had healed her. Great news for her, but meanwhile, Jairus' daughter's life ebbed away. Can you imagine Jairus' frustration and angst?

· · ·

While Jesus was still speaking to the woman, someone else came and told Jairus not to bother Him anymore. His daughter was already dead. Oh, the grief and pain! If the woman hadn't stopped Jesus on the way, maybe He could have healed her. Now, all appeared lost. Jesus told Him, "Do not be afraid any longer, only believe and she will be made well" (Luke 8:50.) Jesus arrived at Jairus's house. The mourners laughed at Jesus when He said she was only asleep. They knew she was dead. Then Jesus took the girl's hand and told her to get up. She arose right before their eyes.

Jesus used the hemorrhaging woman to bring greater glory to Himself, and to help others believe He was the promised Messiah. From Jairus' perspective, the interruption was more than inconvenient. It seemed catastrophic. His daughter was dead. Sick people can get well, but dead people stay dead. If Jesus healed her when she was only sick, they might have merely considered Him a healer. Jesus waited until Jairus' daughter died to show Jairus and all present that He was more than a healer. He is God. He has the power over life and death.

Interruptions never annoyed Jesus. Let's face it, nothing surprised Jesus. He saw interruptions as opportunities to help. The interruptions were His ministry. When injuries interrupt our lives, and especially our training schedules, we should have the same attitude that Jesus did. How would God have us use the time? What can we do to help? How has God gifted us to serve His people? We may find that God uses our injuries to accomplish something we could not have foreseen. I wrote my first book while I was laid up with my plantar fasciitis injury. God used my injury in a way I never could have imagined! This collection of devotional thoughts on running is my fifth book. I'm not saying that if I hadn't been injured, I wouldn't have become an author, but it sped up the process. Now I'm as addicted to writing as I am to running. I still hate injuries, but I'm trying to learn to call them divine appointments. This book is called, "Running for the Glory of God." Sometimes, God can use "not running" for His glory too. How has He done that in your life?

CHAPTER 12

RUNNING IS A LOT LIKE FAITH

HOW IS RUNNING LIKE FAITH? As any runner will tell you, there's no substitute for training. If you're preparing for a half-marathon or marathon, or just want to get in better shape, you have to put in the miles. It is not wise to attempt a long run without proper training! There have been many days when I've had a training run on the calendar that I just didn't feel like running. In Texas, it can be too cold, too hot, too rainy, or too windy. I can be like Goldilocks. I like the weather just right. If I wait for perfect running weather in Texas, I may never run. Other times, I'm just tired and I'd prefer to take the day off. If I really want to get in shape and stay in shape, I don't have the luxury of blowing off runs. I have to get out there and log the miles even when I don't want to. No one else can run them for me.

The same is true of faith. It's been said that God has no grandchildren. That means that God does not grant salvation to people because their parents believe in Jesus. Every person must receive Jesus as Lord and Savior in his or her own life. No one can believe for us. If today were race day, and I haven't put in the miles, I'm going to have an atrocious race. In 2007, I entered the New York City Marathon. I didn't start training until about 10 weeks before the race. I knew I wasn't in marathon shape, but I ran 15 miles a few weeks before, so I thought I could gut out the last 11 miles. Huge mistake! The marathon completely exposed my failure to train. I ran the first 15 miles of the race, but the 59th Street Bridge I mentioned earlier crushed me. I walked most of the last 11 miles. Race day is judgment day. It's when our performance judges our training. If I've trained well, my race results should show it. If I haven't trained, my race will undoubtedly expose that too. There's no hiding from the judgment of the race.

Jesus' return will also be a day of judgment. On that day, Jesus will know our faith or lack of it. As the race judges whether we've trained properly, Jesus judges whether we have believed in Him by faith. We won't be able to pretend we believe when we don't. We won't be able to rely on the faith of others. He knows our hearts. There is no substitute for personal faith. No one can believe for you.

What does it mean to have personal faith in Jesus? It means we acknowledge we are sinners and that our sin disqualifies us from heaven. Our holy God can't allow us into heaven in our sinful condition. But this is where it gets good. Jesus lived the sinless life that we could not live. His sinless life qualified Him to be the perfect sacrifice that God demands for sin. When Jesus died on the cross, He said, "It is finished." He meant He had made the sacrifice that God requires for sin. He paid the price required for each of us to get into heaven. All we have to do is to believe in Him for our salvation. We don't rely on our performance; we rely on His good works. By faith God saves us. When we die, God won't see us in our sin. He will credit us with Jesus's sinless perfection simply because we have believed in Him. The fancy theological word for that is imputation. God imputes or credits Jesus's perfect life to us.

Isn't that amazing?! Runners don't get credit for someone else's miles. We have to run our own. Most things in life are like that. We aren't normally able to receive the benefits for someone else's work. But the benefits of faith are an exception to the rule. Though Jesus did the work, He put in the miles so to speak; we get credit for Jesus' work through faith in Him.

Sometimes I wish running was like that. When the spring rains come, or the Texas sun is blazing in the summer, or it's cold in the winter, I would love to sit on the couch and take credit for someone else's miles. Running will never be like that. No one can impute their miles to me. But because of God's grace and mercy, He gives us a way to overcome our sin problem. We can't do it ourselves. But we can by faith in Jesus who has already done the work for us. Believe and receive credit for the work He's done. Faith in Jesus is the only way.

CHAPTER 13

MY SPIRITUAL VO2 MAX

EVEN THOUGH I'VE been running for most of my life, I'm not "technical" about it. I'm not an analytics nerd. (No offense to analytics nerds!) I was running a while back with a young guy who just started running. He asked me what my maximum heart rate is when I run. I had no idea. He started talking to me about his max heart rate, his VO_2 max, and his aerobic and anaerobic fitness levels. I've heard these terms before, but didn't know what they meant. Then I bought this fancy new Garmin 245 watch. It tracks every breath I take and every move I make. I've learned that VO_2 max is the maximum volume of oxygen (in milliliters) one can consume per kilogram of body weight at maximum performance. I still don't know what that means really, except that it's a measurement of my overall fitness. My Garmin says my present VO_2 max is 47, which it says is "excellent," and in the top 10% for my age and gender. When I first got the watch only two months ago, my VO_2 max was 45, so I'm trending in the right direction.

I suppose I like that my watch can tell me I'm in good shape for my age, but I don't want to become a slave to analytics. I just want to lace up my shoes and go. The only metrics I've ever tracked are distance and time. As technology continues to improve and fitness data becomes so easily available, should I ignore it? Probably not. In thinking it through, the pros outweigh the cons. It's beneficial to wear a device that can evaluate my physical fitness and help me improve.

In fact, I would love a device that could track my spiritual fitness. Unfortunately, there's no device that can measure my spiritual VO_2 max. What is spiritual fitness anyway? There are many definitions of spiritual fitness on the internet. Most talk about how "spirituality" can help us cope with the difficulties of life and help us enjoy life more. I prefer to think of spiritual fitness in terms of my relationship with Jesus. Am I following Him closely or have I been drifting away? Is He the top priority in my life? Am I motivated by bringing Him glory, or am I trying to achieve personal glory by receiving the praise of men? These are critical questions in evaluating spiritual fitness. I think most Christians would say their spiritual fitness could be better. I'll be the first to raise my hand. How can we improve it?

Psalm 139:23-24 says, "Search me, God, and know my heart; Put me to the test and know my anxious thoughts; and see if there is *any* hurtful way in me and lead me in the everlasting way." God is the only one who can give me a spiritual checkup. If I have an ache or pain, or I can't stop coughing, I can't diagnose myself. I don't know what's going on inside me. I need a doctor. Spiritually, I can't trust myself to evaluate my condition. I need God to do it. I can only use my own subjective and biased standards. He examines me with the light of the Holy Spirit who can illumine the sin in my life, so I can root it out. God can lead me in the direction He wants me to go. He can change my heart, develop my character, and help me love and serve Him more. The Holy Spirit increases my spiritual fitness if I will submit to His evaluation.

David asked God to do that in Psalm 139. David committed many atrocious sins in his lifetime. Adultery with Bathsheba and murdering her husband to cover it up are two of his greatest sins recorded in the Bible for all to read. Yet God called David "a man after God's own heart." Why would God call a sinner like David a man after His own heart? Because David sought the Lord. He wanted a closer walk with God. In Psalm 86:11-12, David wrote, "Teach me Your way, Lord; I will walk in Your truth; Unite my heart to fear Your name. I will give thanks to You, Lord my God, with all my heart, And I will glorify Your name forever." Although David was a sinner, he had a heart committed to God. His lifetime spiritual VO_2 Max was off the chart.

We increase our physical VO_2 max by training. There are many workouts designed to increase our oxygen consumption. We'll know we're in better shape even without a fancy watch to measure our VO_2 max. Just by running, we'll be able to feel it. How can we increase our spiritual VO_2 max? The same way, by training. It's simple, but it's not easy. We have to be people after God's own heart. As we continually ask the Holy Spirit to examine us and to address the sins He reveals, He can change us. The harder we seek after Him, the more responsive He will be to us. Before long, as we spend time with Him and serve His people, we won't need a fancy watch to measure our spiritual VO_2 max. We'll never be able to put a number on it, or measure it with human instruments, but we'll know it's increasing because we will love Him more, we'll have greater peace and strive to do His will.

CHAPTER 14

FIFTEEN MINUTES UNTIL THE STARTING GUN

IF YOU RACE, you know the feeling. You're hydrated so you've been to the porta-potty five times. Should you try to go again? Is there enough time? You do some more calf stretches. Touch your toes a few more times. Have a quick chat with the runner next to you. You're just trying to release all your nervous energy while you wait for the next 15 minutes to pass. It's all over but the running now. You've followed your training plan. You've carbo-loaded. While you wait, music plays in the background to get you psyched up. Then the emcee makes a few last-minute announcements and adds a few corny jokes. You're not really listening though. All you want is to hear that starting gun and get running. Ten minutes until the race, now five. They play the national anthem. Now one minute until the gun.

I'm in the habit of arriving at least an hour early before a race. I want to be sure I have plenty of time. Just recently I drove to a race but typed the wrong address into my GPS. I arrived to find nobody there! That's a terrible feeling. I got where I needed to go with some time left to spare, but I don't like to be rushed. The downside of that strategy is that I'm usually ready to run at least 45 minutes before the race begins. That's a lot of time for nervous energy to build up, and nerves make me need the porta-potty.

There's something I both love and hate about that 45-minutes before the race. I hate that those minutes pass so slowly. During that time, I second guess my training, hydration, and food over the last few days. I wonder if I'm over-trained or undertrained for the race. There's just too much time to think. But I love the lead up to the race too. There's a collective excitement and anticipation in the air. It's like that old Heinz ketchup ad that borrowed Carly Simon's song, "Anticipation." A young kid turns the ketchup bottle over, but it's so thick that he has to wait and wait for it to drop from the bottle onto his cheeseburger. Runners know the feeling of pre-race anticipation and anxiety. It doesn't matter if we're fast or slow. For most of us, we're not racing each other, we're challenging ourselves.

Thirty seconds. The butterflies dance in my belly. Finally, the starter fires the gun, and it's go time. I try not to trip over those around me. I find some room and settle into race pace. Now I can relax and execute my race strategy.

Christianity is all about anticipation. Jesus is coming again, just as He promised. The difference is that we know when the race begins. We don't know when Jesus is coming again. Imagine if we did. What if we knew Jesus was coming again next Tuesday at 9 am? Can you imagine the anticipation and excitement? When asked, Jesus said only the Father knows when He will come again. I'm not advocating guessing dates for Jesus' return. No one who's tried it has ever been right! I'm only asking you to imagine what it would be like if we knew He was coming next Tuesday at 9 am. How would our lives change? What would we do with the few days we have left? I hope we would tell as many people as we could. All people will spend eternity somewhere. Those who put their faith in Jesus will be in heaven with God. Those who do not, will be in hell, separated from God forever.

Those who believe would wait for Him in nearly uncontainable excitement. What will He look like? What will He say to us? We only have a vague idea of what heaven might be like. Who can even imagine spending eternity with Jesus? The day of Jesus' second coming is the hope of Christians all over the world. It's the day when Jesus will fulfill all His promises and bring us to our heavenly home. What a day that will be. How thrilling if we knew it was only a few days away!

We don't know when Jesus is coming again. Faithful disciples have lived and died waiting for His return for 2000 years now. Because it's been so long, and because it may not happen in our lifetime, we probably don't have the eager sense of expectation we have 15 minutes before the starting gun of a race. Jesus told His disciples repeatedly to be prepared.

Matthew 24:42-44: "Therefore be on the alert, for you do not know which day your Lord is coming. But be sure of this, that if the head of the house had known at what time of the night the thief was coming, he would have been on the alert and would not have allowed his house to be broken into. For this reason you must be ready as well; for the Son of Man is coming at an hour when you do not think He will."

I like to schedule several races over the upcoming few months. On those days, I know exactly where I will be on the date and time of the race. I'll be tightening my shoelaces one more time, thinking about one more bathroom trip, eager for the race to begin. I don't know where I'll be when Jesus returns, but I want to live with "15 minutes before the starting gun" anticipation every day. Being prepared means I've done all I can to keep my life free from sin and to serve Him as best I can. My heart's desire is for Jesus to say to me, "Well done good and faithful servant." That day will be better than setting a new PR or winning an Olympic gold medal. I'm waiting for it with eager anticipation.

CHAPTER 15

THE WALL AND THE FALL

THERE ARE ONLY two things that scare me when running. Most runners will admit fear of "hitting the wall" in a marathon. It usually happens around 20 miles. Still six miles to go, but there's nothing left in the tank. Six miles is a long way to go with no fuel, cramped muscles, and a discouraged mind. I've hit the wall more than once and I can testify that it's worthy of my fear! The other thing I fear is falling. I've been running for a long time. I'd say that in the last 25 years of running, I've fallen about five times. Usually, it's an elevated sidewalk crack that trips me up. I remember once tripping over a raised sprinkler head. Even a loose shoelace can be a culprit.

The other day I went out for a ten-mile run in very strong Texas winds. The wind has never tripped me before, but it nearly did on this day. In mid-stride, a powerful gust blew my back foot into my front foot, and I stumbled. If you've ever tripped and fallen, you know what it's like. You don't go down immediately. It's like slow-motion as with every stride your body becomes more horizontal than vertical. You're fighting to regain your balance, but all the while, it seems more certain that you're going to face plant. That's what happened to me. I was three steps into the fall. My body felt like it was parallel to the ground. I was looking for a patch of grass to dive on to break my fall.

Don't you find that life is like that sometimes too? You've suffered some unforeseen turn of events, a cancer diagnosis, financial hardship, a broken relationship, or job loss. You're going down, and the best you can hope for is to miss the pavement and find some grass. This life isn't easy. Jesus warned us Christians that we will have trouble in the world. Where can we find comfort and hope when it seems we're about to eat the pavement?

My favorite verses of comfort and hope when my world is falling apart are Isaiah 41:10-13: "Don't be afraid, for I am with you! Don't be frightened, for I am your God! I strengthen you— yes, I help you— yes, I uphold you with my saving right hand! Look, all who were angry at you will be ashamed and humiliated; your adversaries will be reduced to nothing and perish. When you will look for your opponents, you will not find them; your enemies will be reduced to absolutely nothing. For I am the LORD your God, the one who takes hold of your right hand, who says to you, 'Don't be afraid, I am helping you'" (NET).

God doesn't always prevent suffering or stop bad things from happening to us. When He allows us to go through difficult times, it's often because He's trying to teach us something. Maybe we've become too self-reliant, and God needs to remind us *He* is the provider of all good things. Or we've been engaged in some unconfessed sin and God causes us to suffer the consequences, so we'll repent. Other times, it's just a matter of timing. God has something good for us, but we may suffer while we wait for God to prepare us for it, or it for us. For whatever reason, God allows suffering. He uses it for our good and His glory. God loves us. He doesn't allow suffering because

He's an evil tyrant. He's a good and benevolent God who gave His Son on the cross so we could have eternal life with Him. In the Isaiah passage above, God promises to strengthen us and lift us up by His powerful right hand. If you feel like you're about to face-plant into the sidewalk, remember these promises of God.

When I was mid-fall the other day, I had given up saving myself. My brain said, "just find some grass!" Suddenly I was upright again. I can't explain it. It was as if God caught me and stood me up on my two feet again. I don't have another explanation. I was going down, and there were only two options, grass, or pavement. There was a third option I hadn't considered. That God would put me back on my feet with His powerful right hand.

I still fear "the wall" and "the fall," but not enough that I don't run. Runners run. That's what we do. If we hit the wall, we rely on our training and fight through it. If we fall, we shake it off and tend to our injuries when we get home. When we've hit the wall or had a fall in life, we ask God to fulfill His promises to lift us up with His powerful hand. He's sworn to do it. We can trust His promises.

CHAPTER 16

HIS EYE IS ON THE SPARROW

I WAS RUNNING on one of my usual routes recently when I came across this baby bird, lying dead on the sidewalk. I gave him a little nudge, hoping he was only injured and that maybe I could help. No response. My thoughts immediately went to Matthew 10:29-31: "What is the price of two sparrows—one copper coin? But not a single sparrow can fall to the ground without your Father knowing it. And the very hairs on your head are all numbered. So don't be afraid; you are more valuable to God than a whole flock of sparrows" (NLT.)

In this passage, Jesus was teaching His disciples about God's love for His people, and how valuable they are to Him. God cares for all His creatures. Though sparrows have little monetary value—not even one sparrow can fall to the ground without God knowing it and allowing it. Jesus said that if God values and cares for sparrows, how much more will He care for us? It's a rhetorical question. Humanity was God's last and greatest creation. So great that He sent His Son to die to save us. He loves each of us and knows us intimately. He even numbers the hairs on our heads. That's why Jesus instructs us not to be afraid. Each of us is more valuable than an entire flock of sparrows.

But if we're so valuable, why do we suffer hardship in this life and then die? That's the same fate as sparrows. How can Jesus tell us we're more valuable than sparrows when we're all going to die? It's because Jesus loves us much more than birds. If we need proof, it's that Jesus became a man, lived a sinless life, and died on a cross to save us. He did not die to save birds. When He agreed to be born as a human baby, it was so He could experience everything humans experience: temptation, rejection, pain, loss, hunger and even death. In His whole life, He never sinned. Anything we experience, He experienced without sinning.

On the cross, He paid the penalty for our sins, not His own. Pilate pronounced Him not guilty several times, but because of political pressure, sent Him to the cross anyway. This was all part of the plan since before God created us, that Jesus would die for our sins so that whoever believes in Him shall not perish but have eternal life (John 3:16.) God cares for sparrows, just as Matthew 6:26 says: "Look at the birds of the sky, that they do not sow, nor reap, nor gather crops into barns, and yet your heavenly Father feeds them. Are you not much more important than they?" But Jesus did not die for sparrows. He died for you and me.

There's an old gospel hymn called *His Eye Is On the Sparrow*, written in 1905 by lyricist Civilla D. Martin and composer Charles H. Gabriel. Such singers from Whitney Houston to Bill Gaither to George Beverly Shea, performed this song. This is the middle verse:

"Let not your heart be troubled," His tender word I hear,
And resting on His goodness, I lose my doubts and fears;
   though by the path He leadeth, but one step I may see;

His eye is on the sparrow, and I know He watches me;
His eye is on the sparrow, and I know He watches me.

We need not worry about present troubles nor fear death if we're children of God. His eye is even on the sparrow, but He loves you and me. I was sad to see that little bird dead on the sidewalk. But it reminded me of God's unfathomable love for me. Before I saw the bird, my mind was drifting. I usually focus on mundane things like my pace and breathing, and how far I have left in the run. After I saw the bird, I finished my run, thanking God for saving me and providing for me. I trust His promise that even though my body will die, He will bring me safely home into His glorious kingdom.

CHAPTER 17

AN OBNOXIOUS HONKER

WHEN RUNNING up to a busy intersection, I'm always relieved when there are no cars coming. Runners never want to break their stride waiting for cars. I came to an intersection on a recent run, and though there was a car coming from my right in the distance, I could easily cross the street without speeding up. As soon as I stepped into the street, the driver started beeping at me. In eight strides or so, I had finished crossing, but the driver kept honking his horn. I turned my head, thinking maybe the driver recognized me. That wasn't it. He was just extremely angry that he might have to slow down for me. Obviously, the guy was not a runner. Being from the northeast, I'm no stranger to honking. We use our horns more than our turn signals. In the days before Jesus came into my life, I would have given this driver the single finger salute. Now that I've been saved for about twenty years, I just felt sorry for him.

Have you noticed how angry everyone seems to be these days? You can't turn on the news without seeing the hatred people harbor toward each other. The most benign post on social media can quickly turn into name calling. Even on sports talk shows, everyone is always yelling and arguing!! What's going on? The world is in a downward spiral of stress. The Covid-19 pandemic has caused deep divisions. How to cure the virus, whether to get the vaccine, whether the government can require people to get the vaccine, are all political issues that have polarized the nation. We could say the same for political party affiliation, abortion, and Critical Race Theory. The media encourages division because it makes for good news stories. People get riled by the news and then use social media to voice their opinions. Their followers "like" their posts and use gang mentality to shout down anyone brave enough to challenge them. Gone are the days when people could hold different opinions and still be friends. Now, to disagree with someone means to hate them.

One reason I like to run is that it allows me freedom from all that's wrong in the world for a brief time. I put my airpods in and either listen to a sermon, or a podcast about other interests, or just listen to music. Running is an escape. This driver reminded me that no matter how far I run, I can't escape the world. As Christians, we're called to influence the world for good. Two ways to do this come to mind. One is Paul's command in Romans 12:18: "If possible, so far as it depends on you, be at peace with all people. As much as it depends on you, live in peace with all people." That means that we should try not to start a conflict. If we find ourselves in one, we need to do whatever we can to resolve it. Jesus said, "Blessed are the peacemakers, for they will be called sons of God" (Matthew 5:9.)

Peacemaking is more than resolving conflict between ourselves and others. It's avoiding saying or doing things that will start conflict, and it's also resolving disagreements that don't involve us. We may find ourselves in a position to resolve an argument between others. We should help others be at peace with each other. Even more important is to help people know peace with God. Jesus died for the sin of the entire world, but only those who receive the gift through faith will have peace with God. When we tell people about Jesus and lead them to Him, God is using us to make peace between God and man. What an incredible calling.

The other way we can influence the world for good is to remember Jesus' words from the Sermon on the Mount. Love your enemies and pray for those who persecute you (Matthew 5:44.) We may not be able to make peace with everyone. It takes two to tango. If someone won't reconcile, there's no peace, but you can always pray for that person. Leave the results in God's very capable hands.

While we're in the world, Christians must do whatever we can to make it better. They will know we are Christians by our love! Thinking about this obnoxious honker also reminds me of how I long for the world to come. In heaven, no one will honk their horn at me. Temptation to return evil for evil with a crude gesture won't exist. There will be nothing but pure joy as we bask in the savior's love and presence. I admit, most of this did not immediately come to my mind when the driver repeatedly honked at me. To be honest, my immediate reaction was to ask God to smite the obnoxious honker with fire and brimstone! It takes what I would call "sanctified reflection" to put myself in that person's shoes. Maybe he wasn't supposed to work that day, but the boss made him come in. Maybe he just had a fight with his wife or has a sick child. It's possible he was just a jerk, but if I give him the benefit of the doubt, I can give him grace. No matter the reason he honked, I can still pray for him. When it happened, I only had about a half mile left on my run. I was mad that he interrupted my peace and thought about it the rest of the way home. I didn't pray for him then, but I'm praying for him now. When Jesus said to pray for our enemies, I think that's what He meant. Pray for their salvation.

I wouldn't recognize the obnoxious honker if I saw him on the street. But God knows him! Maybe because I ran that day, and because God put me in the path of a driver having a bad morning, and because I prayed for him, maybe God will use all those circumstances to bring him to saving faith. That's what I call running for the glory of God!

CHAPTER 18

CARBO-LOADING

AS I WRITE THIS, I'm planning to run a race called the Frisco Running Company half-marathon in McKinney, TX tomorrow. As any runner knows, lots of carbs and water are the dietary fare for the days leading up to a long race. I don't mind that at all. I could live on good bread (a hard to find delicacy in Texas), pasta, cereal, potatoes and rice. Scientists and dieticians say carbo loading maximizes our muscles' ability to store glycogen, which converts to energy during the race. Studies confirm that runners filled with glycogen perform better on race day than those who skip the carbs. So today, I'll be looking for opportunities to fill my belly (and muscles) with rice, pasta, and excellent bread, if I can find any. Tomorrow morning, I'll eat an English muffin and an egg, and be off to the race. To do my best, I need my glycogen storage fully maximized.

Smart runners don't neglect the carbo-load. It's the last piece of the training puzzle. If you've spent months putting in the countless miles on the road, through pain, loneliness, rain, or freezing cold, you won't disregard the fuel you need on race day. Many of the big races also host a pasta party the night before. Proper fuel is a necessity to run well.

Christians have access to fuel that empowers our walk with Christ. I'm talking about the infinite power of the Holy Spirit that enables us to become more like Jesus. Every person who has received Jesus as Savior is a Christian, and every Christian has the Holy Spirit living inside of him. The Holy Spirit is not a force or an energy like carbs are to a runner. The Holy Spirit is a person: the third person of the Trinity, God the Father, Jesus the Son, and the Holy Spirit. They are all God and yet God is one. Theologians say that God is one in essence and three in person. It's very hard for our finite minds to understand, but that doesn't make it any less true.

Each member of the Trinity has distinct roles beyond glorifying each other for all eternity. The Holy Spirit has many roles. In Acts 1:8, Jesus said, "you will receive power when the Holy Spirit comes upon you." The Holy Spirit inspired the authors of the Bible to write the scriptures. (2 Peter 1:20-21) He helps to illuminate the scriptures to us so we can understand them and apply them to our lives (1 Corinthians 2:9-10.) He helps us remember what we have read and studied (John 16:12-13.) He prays for us (Romans 8:26-27) and produces the character of Jesus in us. Galatians 5:22-23 calls these character traits the "fruit of the Spirit." The Holy Spirit teaches us to look different and be different from the rest of the unbelieving world. Through His power, our attitudes and behaviors become more like Jesus', and less like our old selves.

In "The Four Priorities," a book by Dr. John Tolson and Larry Kreider, the authors tell the story of Ira Yates, a man who owned a sheep ranch in West Texas during the Great Depression. He couldn't earn enough money to survive and ended up on government assistance. Later, scientists and an oil company crew detected that there might be oil under his land. Yates gave them permission to dig, and they struck oil, lots of oil. He became a multi-millionaire nearly overnight. Yates owned the oil on the day he bought the land. He just didn't know the oil was beneath it. The moral of the story? Too many Christians are living below the poverty level spiritually when they have access to the greatest riches available in the power of the Holy Spirit. [1]

How do we access this power? Just like we have to eat carbs for them to affect our performance, we have to be filled with the Holy Spirit too (Ephesians 5:18.) We do this through encountering Him through prayer and Bible study. The power of the Holy Spirit is available to any Christian who seeks His guidance and asks for help. The Holy Spirit's role is always to glorify Jesus and to point us to Him. Since the Holy Spirit is God, He cannot fail in His role. However, we need to cooperate with Him. The Bible says we can grieve the Spirit (Ephesians 4:30), and quench the Spirit (1 Thessalonians 5:19.) That means we can choke out His power by ignoring Him, or by continual sin. The Bible also says the Holy Spirit can fill us and lead us if we submit to His authority.

I like the concept of filling. It corresponds well to my carbo-loading illustration. Fill ourselves with carbs to perform well on race day. That's why I'm stuffed full of carbs today. Be filled with the Holy Spirit to live more holy lives and bear more fruit for the kingdom of God. The awesome power that raised Jesus from the grave is available to us! The Holy Spirit maximizes our Christian lives as carbs maximize our race performance. If you're a Christian, you already have the Holy Spirit living inside you. Why grieve or quench Him? Instead, fill yourself with Him and watch God change your life in new incredible ways.

CHAPTER 19

STRENGTH FROM WEAKNESS

AND NOW FOR a post-race report from the Frisco Running Company half-marathon. Sometimes you have it and sometimes you don't. It was 23 degrees when the race started. That's bitter cold by Texas standards, even in January. It wasn't the cold though; it was me. I wouldn't change anything I did before the race. I trained properly, ate the right foods, drank lots of water, and even though my time was decent, I never felt comfortable through the race. It was a battle from start to finish. If I've learned anything in my running life, it's that although proper preparation increases the likelihood of excellent results, it's no guarantee. The problem is human weakness, more specifically, my own weakness. My human body has so many limitations.

When I run, I often thank God for giving me the strength to keep pounding the pavement. I was born in 1965. You do the math; I'm not a young man anymore. I know there are many people my age who can't run for a variety of reasons, so I give thanks. At the same time, running reminds me every day that I completely depend on God for every breath I take. When my lungs are burning and my legs feel like cinder blocks, that's God reminding me of my human limitations. When I'm in the last mile of a race and have almost nothing left in the tank, I often think of Paul's words in 2 Corinthians 12.

Paul had a "thorn in his flesh" as he described it. We don't know what it was, but some malady he also described as "a messenger from Satan to torment me, to keep me from exalting myself." Paul prayed three times for God to remove it. God always answers prayer, but sometimes the answer is "no." God said to Paul, "My grace is sufficient for you, for my power is perfected in weakness" (ESV.) God meant that though Paul's physical ailment would remain, the spiritual power of God's grace *is* (present tense) always available.

The weaker the human vessel, the more obvious that God's power is working through that person. So it was with Paul. Other than Jesus, no Christian ever endured more hardship while working tirelessly to bring the gospel to the world. In 2 Corinthians 11, he described being beaten, stoned, shipwrecked, adrift at sea, in danger from robbers, and false brothers, without food and water, and left out in the cold without shelter. What kept Paul going? The grace of the Lord Jesus Christ that was sufficient for Him.

The sufficiency of the grace of Jesus means that no matter what we've done wrong, God will always forgive us if we place our trust in Jesus for forgiveness of our sins. We just ask for forgiveness and God gives us Jesus' righteousness while charging Jesus with our sins. That's the best deal ever! His grace saves us, but it also sustains us. That's why Paul wrote the verse in the present tense. How often have we felt so discouraged that we didn't know how we could make it through the day? Yet we made it through the day because of God's grace and His power carrying us, when we couldn't make it on our own.

Many of you may be familiar with the poem, "Footprints." In it, a man noticed that during the hardest times in his life, he only saw one set of footprints in the sand. He asked God why He left him during these times, when at other times he saw two sets of footprints. God answered that he saw only one set of footprints, not because God left him during those most difficult times, but because God carried Him. That's God's power perfected in our human weakness.

Back to the race. My body begged me to stop. If there had been any spectators braving the freezing temperatures to watch, they would have testified to my human weakness. Somehow, God gave me the strength to finish. He fortified my mind with encouragement that the finish line was only a few minutes away. Then my mind willed my body to finish. I take no credit for it. I give all glory to God to help me do what I would not have been able to do in my power. Obviously, God gives us this power to survive more than just a race. He gives us this power to survive life.

So how can we apply the lesson of God making strength from weakness to our everyday lives? Maybe you're a mother of young kids and the monotony of life seems unbearable. Perhaps you've lost a loved one and you don't know how you can go on without them. Maybe you've just received an ominous diagnosis, or lost your job, or your boss skipped you for a promotion. You might have a conflict with someone that's causing you enormous stress and there's no viable solution. Whatever it is, God says, "My grace is sufficient for you. My power is made perfect in weakness."

When I'm running and about out of gas, I try to think about how I'll feel ten minutes after the race, and not how I feel at that moment. I picture myself breathing normally with a medal around my neck that calls me a "finisher." There may even be junk food to eat at the finish line, so I imagine myself eating cookies, pizza, or a donut. The point is not to focus on the present pain, but the future reward. I'm not minimizing the pain of life. I'm only suggesting that it becomes more bearable if we focus on the "after" rather than the "during." Heaven is forever! We are weak. God is strong. Admit your need for Jesus and receive strength you never knew existed. God promises us the crown of life for finishing the race well. That's better than the best donut you've ever eaten!

CHAPTER 20

CHASING KIDS

ONE OF MY regular running routes takes me past the local elementary school. Since I run early in the morning, I usually see lots of kids. The other day, a mom parked her car a couple blocks away from the school to avoid the mayhem of crossing guards directing traffic. She let her three kids out of the car, and they began their walk through the park with mom to the school. I came up behind them soon after and passed them. These three kids couldn't have been older than 7. They weren't going to allow an old man to pass them. They took off like a shot and ran as fast as they could until they were about 20 yards ahead of me. Then their burning lungs gave out. They stopped and put their hands on their knees gasping for air. As I passed them, I smiled and waved. I run at about 8:45 pace. I'm not the fastest guy in the world, but not the slowest either. My motto is, "a sure and steady pace finishes the race."

Slow and steady is the motto for many things in life. Investing and wealth accumulation, climbing the corporate ladder if that's what you're into, weight loss, you name it, there are very few things worth doing that we can do quickly. Our spiritual growth is similar. Someone said, "when God wants to grow a mushroom, He takes 6 hours. When He wants to grow an oak tree, He takes 60 years." I would add, "When He wants to make a mature Christian, He takes a lifetime." When I first became a Christian, I devoured the Bible and many other Christian books. It was all so new to me, and I was learning and growing in knowledge by leaps and bounds. Still, knowledge does not equal wisdom or experience.

We gain wisdom through knowledge and experience, and it's often a long process. The fancy theological word for spiritual growth is "sanctification." It means "to be holy or set apart." Included in the word's meaning is the lifelong progression of becoming more like Christ. Sanctification is God's Holy Spirit working in us to make us more like Jesus. Phil. 1:6 says: "He (God) who began a good work in you will carry it on to completion in the day of Christ Jesus."

However, the process of sanctification also requires us to cooperate with the Holy Spirit as He molds us and shapes us into the image of Jesus. For example, 1 Thessalonians 4:3-5 says: "It is God's will that you should be sanctified: that you should avoid sexual immorality; that each of you should learn to control your own body in a way that is holy and honorable, not in passionate lust like the pagans, who do not know God." We have a choice in our behavior.

Sanctification is the Holy Spirit working through us. We allow the Holy Spirit to change us to become more like Jesus. I came to faith later in life and I am abundantly aware that I am a sinner. It seems like it would take 10 lifetimes to make me more like Jesus. There's no reason to worry about how long it will take to become more like Jesus. We'd only get discouraged and give up because imitating Jesus perfectly is an impossible goal. We just need to focus on sure and steady pace to finish the race. Since we'll never model Jesus's life perfectly, how can we measure spiritual growth? The only way I know is to compare ourselves to how we were 6 months ago, a year ago, or 5 years ago. Can we forgive others more easily now than we would have then? Are we praying more and listening for God's voice more effectively now than we did then? Do we focus more on others now than we did then?

We've all heard the expression, "It's not a sprint, it's a marathon." Runners know the truth of that phrase better than anyone. To us, it's not a saying, it's a reality of our lives. Most people use the phrase as a figure of speech to describe the process of growth and change. If people are being kind to us, they use that phrase to encourage us when we fail to meet a deadline, make a mistake parenting our kids, or lose our cool waiting for hours on the customer service line at Walmart! Sometimes progress is two steps forward and one step back. If that's the case, we've still made one step forward. That's progress. Let's not allow slow growth to discourage us. Slow growth is still growth. God knows where He wants to take us, and He can get us there.

As these kids ran by me, I had a good laugh. I knew they couldn't hold that pace for more than a few seconds. They'll never remember this story that I'm telling you, but over the course of their childhood, they will learn they can only run at full speed for so long. They will learn that if they want to run farther, they'll have to run slower. That's a lesson for all Christians. We shouldn't allow frustration to stop us when we set goals and then fall or fail. Having the gumption to try should encourage us. When we think over the events of the day with regret because we could have handled a situation better, remember and believe that God will give us another chance to make it right. He knows where we are weak.

Patience is something I need to work on. When I fail, I know God will put other opportunities in my path until I begin to get it right. He gives me lots of opportunities because I fail all the time, especially in my car! Don't focus on the one failure. Focus on the successes. Remember that a sure and steady pace finishes the race. Adjust your strategy for growth and try again. Then keep trying until you finish. Our faith grows and strengthens not through quick and easy success, but through failure, perseverance, and endurance. These are necessary tools in every successful runner's toolbox, and are just as important for the long, slow run to Christlikeness.

CHAPTER 21

THE FIRST MILE

I'VE LEARNED over the years not to judge a run by the first mile. I'm sure you runners know what I mean. On most runs, I feel various aches and pains in the first mile. My breathing and stride aren't quite right. It takes a while to get warmed up and into a rhythm. For these reasons, the first mile is always my slowest, at least 30 seconds slower than my second mile on average. To go from standing still to race pace is a jolt to my body. My brain has told my body to move, but my body is still fighting what Newton called the laws of motion. Newton's first law of motion states that an object stays at rest unless acted upon by an outside force. My body wants to stay at rest all the time. But the force acting against it is my brain telling my body to move! My body reluctantly obeys, but it takes a while to get up to speed. Most days, if I let my body have its way, I'd stop before I finished the first mile. I wouldn't accomplish much in running or racing if I let my body rule my mind. I've learned if I just keep my body moving, eventually it will catch up to my brain, and we can all have a pleasant run together!

· · ·

The concept of difficult beginnings is familiar to runners and non-runners alike. If your family moved when you were a kid and you had to start at a new school, it took a while before you made friends and felt at home. When you went to college, or began a new job, it's usually about a year before you feel comfortable. What about the first year of marriage? Counselors say most couples who come for help are in their first year of marriage. When God takes two selfish sinners and puts them together under one roof, of course there's going to be an adjustment period. But we shouldn't judge the likelihood of success of a marriage in the first year. Newlyweds usually just have to adjust to a new lifestyle.

In the Bible, God gave plenty of examples of people who had difficult beginnings but turned out just fine. Abraham lied about Sarah being his wife twice but became the model of faith by obeying God and being willing to sacrifice his son Isaac (Genesis 22.) Jacob was a liar and scammer early in his life, but God changed him after wrestling with him at Peniel (Genesis 32:32-33.) Jacob became a man of faith and the father of the twelve tribes of Israel. Moses had a stutter before God called him to lead the Jews out of Egypt (Exodus 4:10.) David started out as the runt of seven sons before being anointed king of Israel (1 Sam. 16.)

I didn't become a Christian until my mid-thirties. I did so many things that bring me shame and hurt me or others. But it's not how you start, it's how you finish that matters. I look at those years like I look at the first mile of a run. It's behind me now and I can't change it. I have to keep moving forward in the love and grace of Jesus. Like struggling through the first mile until my body falls into sync with my mind; becoming a new person after a hard start is an act of the will through the power of the Holy Spirit. 2 Corinthians 5:17 says: "Therefore, if anyone is in Christ, the new creation has come. The old has gone, the new is here!" We become new creations when we believe the gospel and the Holy Spirit comes to dwell in our bodies. He gives us the power to change.

Ephesians 4:22-24 says: "You were taught, with regard to your former way of life, to put off your old self, which is being corrupted by its deceitful desires; to be made new in the attitude of your minds; and to put on the new self, created to be like God in true righteousness and holiness" (NIV.) My favorite passage on becoming a new person despite a tough start is Romans 6:11-12: "In the same way, count yourselves dead to sin but alive to God in Christ Jesus. Therefore, do not let sin reign in your mortal body so that you obey its evil desires" (NIV.)

Have you had a hard start in life? Do you have regrets that bring you shame and hurt others? We all do. We've all blown it many times. The good news is that the first mile doesn't have to define our race. Life really is a marathon not a sprint. Jesus gives us all the grace we could ever need. He forgives all our sins, even the ones we haven't committed yet. When we fail, He says to us, "You're forgiven. I already paid for that sin on the cross. Go in peace." The power of the indwelling Holy Spirit allows us to change. Perhaps better said, He *causes* us to change. The Holy Spirit is God Himself, and He doesn't want to live in a dirty house. He'll work hard to clean us up. We just need to cooperate.

If you're disappointed with your start. Don't give up. The Holy Spirit is powerful! He can shape our will. Our wills train our minds. Our minds control our bodies. When we get this worked out, everything will be in sync, working in harmony together with the will of God. In the beginning, just like at the start of a run, our bodies will fight our minds. But the longer we stick with it, the more we find that our bodies, minds, and wills agree, and we can all enjoy the run together, pleasing God and glorifying Him with our lives.

CHAPTER 22

GETTING LOST

IN APRIL 2021, I ran in the Irving Marathon. It was my first marathon in over 10 years. I had run a few half-marathons leading up to the Irving Marathon but hadn't completed a full marathon training program. Still, I felt confident that I could run the distance. The start of the race was like most other starts, lots of anxiety until the gun went off, then jostling and positioning until I could settle into a comfortable pace. The first 10 miles went by with no problem. I saw my wife along the course, which is always a great encouragement. I wasn't paying attention to the course as I passed her and missed a turn. It wasn't that big of a deal. She saw it happen and immediately called me on the phone to tell me to turn back. Thank God I had the ringer on. I turned around and got back on track. I wish I could say that was my last misadventure in the race.

The course was a 12 mile "out and back" with a loop on the end. Racers run it twice to finish the race. I noticed I had a problem when I passed the 15-mile mark, but I hadn't even run 13 miles yet. To this day, I don't know how I did it, but at the end of the first out and back, I skipped the loop. I'm sure I wasn't paying attention and missed a sign. It's easy to miss signs when you're dragging and looking at your shoes while running! By the time I figured out what I had done, I was already near the 16-mile mark, way too far to go back and run the loop. I knew my error disqualified me from the race because I hadn't crossed the chip tracker at mile 13. What to do? Should I just walk off the course or keep running? I've never quit a race, so I kept running; but that mishap took all the wind out of my sails. I felt lousy physically and was very upset about being disqualified after running 16 miles. I kept going, planning to get near the finish line and then keep running up and down the street until my watch said I'd run 26.2 miles. Then I'd cross the finish line.

Getting lost is extremely frustrating during a race. I ran 26.2 miles and wasn't an "official" marathon finisher. Life constantly presents learning experiences. Races are not the only places where we can get lost. Sometimes we get lost on our faith journey. I can remember many times when I thought I was on the path that God had for me, but then made one poor decision, one wrong turn, and got off course. That can happen if we're running out ahead of God and not waiting for His perfect timing. It can happen when we're trying to do something God hasn't prepared for us yet. The trick, just as in running a race, is to pay attention to the signs and follow them!

When I knew God wanted us to sell our house in New Jersey and move to Texas to go to seminary, I did everything I could to expedite the sale. I wanted to be in Texas the next week! Timing is everything though. God wanted us to move, but apparently not immediately. We put our house on the market but couldn't find the right buyer for almost two years! I felt lost, confused, and angry with God. I grumbled incessantly, "God, if you want us to move, why won't you bring us a buyer?!" My patience was at its end. I had become very discouraged and probably even depressed. I was like a madman pestering our realtor to hold more open houses to drum up interest. My problem was that I didn't see the signs God was showing me. He was saying, "Yes, I want you to sell your house and move to Texas, but not yet."

I now realize that a quick move would have been extremely traumatic to my family and my law practice. It would take time to get things in order and to prepare for a major move across the country with two kids in grammar school and an ongoing business. God knew it, but I didn't. In retrospect, I can see Him shaking His head lovingly at me. I can almost hear Him say, "Do you not believe I can sell this house in one minute when the time is right?" I couldn't see it then because I thought I had heard from God clearly that He wanted us to move, and then He erected obstacles so we couldn't. We had a great plan, but God's plan is always better than ours. Once God was ready for us to move, He provided a lovely family who appreciated our house as much as we did.

We moved to Texas about two years later than we planned; but we were back on course, according to God's timing, not our own. God knows much more than we do! He's the author of the future. When Jesus stooped down to wash His disciples' feet, He said in John 13:7, "What I am doing you do not understand now, but you will know after this." When we're lost, confused, and don't understand, we need to learn to trust God. We may not understand now, but we will later. The lesson is that it is good to make plans, but we must allow God into the planning process, or we will soon end up lost in confusion, not understanding what to do next. God can bring us where He wants us to go, but it's always best if it's in His time.

In my race, when I neared the finish line, I had only run about 23 miles. The race volunteers signaled for me to turn and cross the finish line, but I ran past them. They yelled for me to come back, but I wouldn't accept a finisher's medal without running 26.2 miles. I found the loop that I missed my first time around the course and ran it then. I crossed the finish line having run a full 26.2 miles, just not in the right order!

I met my wife at the finish. I was disappointed at how the race went, but at least I wasn't lost anymore. A few months later I ran a half marathon on the same course. This time there were no loops; only one out and back. I was very careful. I ran all the miles in the correct order! Sometimes it's as simple as keeping my eyes up and paying attention to the signs.

CHAPTER 23

SAVED BY RUNNING

I HAD lunch with a good friend of mine who's also a member of our church congregation. We got talking about running, and he said that he used to be a runner too. When he was in his 30s, he injured his fascia tendon and had to have surgery. During the pre-op testing and procedures, the doctors discovered a growth in his colon. They told my friend that if they didn't remove this tumor, it would metastasize and kill him. They took out about a foot of his colon, and he's been fine since. He's now in his 80s and has lived a long and Christ-centered life. All because he hurt himself running 50 years ago. He can truthfully say that running, and his injury, saved his life.

Most don't have such dramatic testimonies of how running saved our lives, or do we? I couldn't point to a single event like my friend, but I can reflect on many ways that running has been a lifesaver. Running relieves my stress. Since stress causes high blood pressure, which can lead to heart attacks and stroke, running is an investment in living longer and more productively. As a weight bearing exercise, running also helps build strong bones and strengthen muscles. It improves cardiovascular fitness. It burns calories so I can enjoy fun foods while still maintaining a healthy weight. All these benefits keep me alive and healthy and help me enjoy my life.

I've read somewhere, probably in an article written by a cynic, that running only increases your life by the time you spent running. I'm sure his point was, "I don't want the extra time if it's only time spent running." The author assumes that time spent running is miserable time, so why bother? I'm not aware of any test studies on this theory, but I disagree with the premise. Time spent running is not miserable, but restorative. If I run in the morning, it gets my mind right to face the day. If I run in the middle of the day, it's a break from whatever I'm working on, a chance to clear my mind, and for the creative juices to flow. Every chapter in this book has originated from an idea that came to me while running. The benefits of running are not only physical, but spiritual and emotional as well.

I believe running will increase the length of my life, but I don't run to extend the quantity of my life, but the quality. I'm a member of various running groups on Facebook. My favorite is the "runners over 50" group. I love to get inspiration from people my age and significantly older, who still lace 'em up, and hit the road. I see runners in their 80s still competing at high levels and still living productive lives. They attribute it to running. All I'm doing is following their footsteps. I know it's possible that I could have a stroke, heart attack, or an injury or accident that stops me from running, but I'm going to keep going while I can. When we stop moving, we start dying.

I have no fear of death because I know where I'm going. It's just that while I'm living, I want to live productively. Moses was still working in his 80s. Elijah worked until the day the Lord took him away in a chariot of fire. Paul worked until the day Nero executed him. I take my inspiration from these heroes of the Bible. The ministries God gave them required them to be in good health and able to walk for hundreds of miles. Moses crossed the Red Sea and walked through the wilderness for 40 years. Elijah walked all over Israel doing ministry before God took him up to heaven. Paul traveled thousands of miles on foot, spreading the gospel wherever he went. I don't know what God has planned for me, but I don't want to limit His options by neglecting my body.

Paul wrote in 1 Corinthians 9:26-27: "Therefore I run in such a way as not to run aimlessly; I box in such a way, as to avoid hitting air; but I strictly discipline my body and make it my slave, so that, after I have preached to others, I myself will not be disqualified." He used several athletic metaphors, but the running metaphor is on point. Running was a metaphor for his Christian ministry. His running was not aimless. It had a purpose. It was to make converts and turn them into disciples. His general health and fitness allowed God to use him where physically or spiritually weaker men would have failed. His discipline and training allowed him to "run" the race God had for him so he would not be disqualified. The word that Paul used for "disqualified" could mean "unapproved." In Romans 1:28 and Titus 1:16 he used the same word to describe the unsaved. In this context, he means he trained his body to do the work that God called Him to, so when his race when done, God would approve of his work. His training "saved" him for God's purposes.

In a way, running has saved you and me for the work God has for us to do. We should not take our health for granted. I'm friends with people in that runners over 50 group who lament that they can't run anymore because of various injuries or life circumstances. It's tragic because they want to be out on the road, but they face long rehab stints, or have injuries that will prevent them from ever running again. For as long as God allows, let's keep putting one foot in front of the other to achieve the purposes He has for our lives. We must keep going! We have work to do!

CHAPTER 24

RUNNER'S HIGH

RUNNER'S high is a feeling many runners experience during or after a run. The brain causes this feeling of elation or euphoria by releasing hormones called endorphins. This massive endorphin rush activates the part of your brain that releases dopamine, a feel-good chemical. The combination of the endorphin and dopamine release causes a runner's high. [1]

I experienced runner's high on a recent 15k in Dallas. I'm accustomed to running half marathons, but 15k is a little shorter, so I tried to increase my typical half-marathon pace. For the first 4 miles, I averaged about 8:15 miles. That's fast for me: but I felt great, so I put the pedal down. It was around mile 7 that I noticed this euphoric feeling, like I could run like this all day, and nothing could stop me. I haven't experienced runner's high very often, so initially I didn't recognize it. Eventually, it hit me. I'm in the middle of a runner's high! I ran each of the last five miles under 8 minutes, with the fastest mile at 7:33. For me, that's really fast.

. . .

Some runners say they experience it all the time. Others say they never have. I could probably count on two hands the number of times I've felt it. Now that I have, I crave it! That high can become very addicting. People who don't run think runners are crazy. My running friends know there's nothing like the runner's high. People pay thousands of dollars on illegal drugs for what we get for free!

Experts say runner's high usually happens when running at 70-85% of maximum intensity. That pushes the body into a state of stress, which releases the chemicals that cause runner's high. Running for one to two hours is usually the zone for runner's high. Experts say we should run consistently to stay in good enough shape to experience it. Adding high-speed intervals to workouts keeps your body from adjusting to a certain level of activity. High intensity intervals of short duration may increase the stress factor causing the body to mass produce endorphins. A final trick is to try not to think about achieving runner's high. Just zone out and let it come naturally. [2]

Runners never know if or when they will experience runner's high and it doesn't last forever. Christians know a similar feeling. It's not a physical high, but a spiritual high. Jesus said in John 10:10: "I came that they may have life and have it abundantly." The Greek word for "abundant" means "exceedingly, beyond measure, a quantity so abundant as to be considerably more than what one would expect." Jesus came so we could have that kind of abundant joy. Our abundant life begins the moment we receive Jesus Christ as Lord and Savior. From that moment, we have eternal life that we can never lose. Jesus defined eternal life in John 17:3: "Now this is eternal life: that they may know you, the only true God, and Jesus Christ, whom you have sent." One key then to the euphoric spiritual joy is knowing God and Jesus personally, and that we have eternity in heaven as our destination. That brings joy despite our circumstances; a joy we can never lose.

But what about today? If our only joy is the promise of heaven in the future while we endure this hard life, we are completely missing the picture. Jesus said in John 5:24: "'Truly, truly, I say to you, he who hears My word, and believes Him who sent Me, has eternal life, and does not come into judgment, but has passed out of death into life." Eternal life does not begin when we die, it begins the moment we believe. Believers already have it. We've passed out of death and into eternal life *now*, and Jesus wants us to enjoy eternal life *now*. Joy is not necessarily in long life, health, wealth, or status. Jesus never promised those things. Euphoric joy comes from knowing God and knowing Jesus Christ. It comes from knowing today that we're saved for all eternity. It comes from living free from guilt or fear, even when the circumstances of life are hard. Because of Jesus's death and resurrection, we're free to live a life pleasing to Him and to ourselves.

I've never been more joyful than I am right now. I know I'm saved and free to fulfill God's purposes for my life. He's given me a flock of believers to shepherd. For the last five years, I've known without a doubt that I'm doing what God designed and called me to do. I could not say that about the first 50 years of my life. Now, I have euphoric joy over my eternity and my present. Beyond that, I have a great family, and as of now I'm in very good health. What else could anyone ask? That's not to say I don't suffer hardship like anyone else. Even in my darkest days when I was so depressed I could barely move, I still knew that God loved me, and Jesus died for me. When you have the joy, joy, joy, joy down in your heart, not even suffering can take that from you.

. . .

I will keep running as long as my body allows. I'll crawl out of bed for Saturday morning long runs, add in high-intensity interval training, and run lots of races, chasing that elusive runner's high. Hopefully, I'll feel it again. But even if I don't, I'll live out my life enjoying the spiritual high of knowing Jesus, knowing I'm in His will and that He's using me for His purposes. I want this spiritual high for you too!

CHAPTER 25

A MATTER OF PERSPECTIVE

IT'S FEBRUARY IN DALLAS, and we're in the middle of a cold spell. I'm not looking for sympathy from runners who live in the north. Y'all regularly run in temperatures well below o. I don't envy you. But no one's making you live there either! Here, a cold spell means in the 20s with wind chills in the teens or single digits. We're expecting sleet and freezing rain starting later today and throughout tomorrow. Since we don't plow, salt, or sand the streets here, it will be nearly impossible to run on ice coated roads tomorrow. I looked at my marathon training schedule, and it didn't allot for two straight days of rest. I'm training for an April marathon, so I had to get out this morning for 6 miles.

I have a route that brings me back to the house every three miles for water. I started out running with the wind at my back, and it wasn't bad at all. But then I knew the dreaded turn around was coming when I would run into a headwind. Falling ice crystals pelted my face like tiny needles. It was a relief to finish the second loop and get home. Some of you cold weather runners will think I'm a wimp for complaining about what might seem like a spring day to you. Others of you will think I'm crazy for even going out in such weather. It all depends on your perspective.

When Jesus walked the earth 2000 years ago, He met people who fell at His feet in worship and others who plotted to kill Him. It was all a matter of their perspective. Many of the regular folks had been waiting for their promised Messiah their entire lives. Jesus checked many of the boxes. He was born in Bethlehem as Micah 5:2 prophesied. Jesus was born of a virgin as Isaiah 7:14 prophesied. He descended from the line of David and of Judah. When He spoke, it was with great authority, not like their religious leaders. He healed many sick people, as Isaiah prophesied. From the perspective of regular people whom Jesus loved and helped, it would be easy to believe Jesus could be the Messiah.

Then there's the perspective of the religious leaders, the scribes, Pharisees, and Sadducees. Jesus was not one of them. They saw Him as a lawbreaker and a threat to their power and position. Jesus healed on the Sabbath and told those He healed to get up and carry their mats home. The leaders considered carrying a mat "work," which was prohibited on the Sabbath. Jesus challenged everything they taught about the Scriptures. He told them their hunger to be admired by the people and to keep their authority and high standing in the community skewed their perspective of the scriptures. On top of all that, the people were following Jesus rather than them. The leaders hated Jesus and wanted Him dead. From their perspective, Jesus was not the Messiah, but a blasphemer and a heretic. It's all a matter of perspective.

Two-thousand years later, we have the New Testament in our hands. We know how the story ended. The scribes, Pharisees, and Sadducees succeeded in having Jesus killed. But He rose again on the third day. Then He walked on earth again with His disciples for another 40 days before ascending into heaven. What's left for us to decide is our perspective about Jesus. Is He the Son of God, the second person of the Trinity, the One who died for our sin so we might have eternal life? That's who He claimed to be. The evidence supports His claim. Who else could turn water into wine, five loaves and two fish into a meal for 5000, heal blindness and leprosy, raise the dead, and rise from the dead Himself?

The other perspective is that He was not the Messiah, the savior of the world. That perspective can take many forms. Some people admire Him as a great man, or ethical teacher, but refuse to believe that He was God. Other people continue to believe that He was a heretic or a crazy person. After all, who would claim to be God and then allow Himself to be crucified if He was powerful enough to stop it? Non-believers fall into lots of camps, but the one thing they all have in common is the perspective that Jesus was not the one true God, did not die for their sins, did not rise from the dead, and they owe Him no allegiance or obedience.

In Matthew 16:14-17, Jesus asked the apostles who the people said He was. They answered, "Some say John the Baptist; and others, Elijah; and still others, Jeremiah, or one of the other prophets." He said to them, "But who do you yourselves say that I am?" Simon Peter answered, "You are the Christ, the Son of the living God." And Jesus said to him, "Blessed are you, Simon Barjona, because flesh and blood did not reveal this to you, but My Father who is in heaven."

Peter got it right. What's your perspective? Jesus made outrageous claims; claims made by no one else who ever lived. He performed miracles that no one had ever seen. Jesus proved He could control nature, by calming the raging sea. He showed His power over sickness and demons several times so the people said things like, "We've never seen anything like this."

He even showed His power over death by raising others from the dead and then raising Himself. Do you believe Jesus is who He said He is? If not, why not? What further proof would satisfy you? Or are you putting off a decision until a later time? These are serious questions any nonbeliever should ask. The consequences are eternal.

I'm friends with a guy on Facebook who's in his late 60s who runs over 100 miles a week. Every single week! From my perspective, that's just flat out crazy! Who can do that? And why? I'm more of a 20-30 mile a week runner. To some, that's nothing. To others, that's more than they've run in their lives. Whether we run 100 miles a week, 20 miles, or zero miles won't affect our eternity. Runners run because it makes us happy and healthy. However, what we believe about Jesus makes all the difference for our eternity. Everyone has a choice about where they will spend eternity. Those who don't believe in Jesus will spend eternity separated from Him. But those who trust Him for salvation, will spend eternity in heaven with Him. It's really just a matter of perspective.

CHAPTER 26

RACE VOLUNTEERS

VOLUNTEERS ARE essential to the success of any race. They're needed to set up the start and finish lines, organize race packet pickup, stand on the course to direct runners like me who are prone to getting lost, and distribute water during the race and medals after. They're at the race site long before the runners arrive to set up and stay long after for take down. That's only scratching the surface of all they do. Yet volunteering for races is a thankless job. Runners typically take them for granted. Volunteers are nameless, faceless folks, who serve us. Service is a humble task with no glory in it for the volunteer. No one cheers for them. They get no finisher's medal, no name listed in the race results, no stories of how well they ran, and no paycheck. Why do they do it?

There's surely a social aspect. It's fun to hang around with people and cheer on the runners. Sometimes volunteers come in groups. A whole family, office, book club, or running club might work a race together. The New York Road Runners Club entices people to volunteer by giving them entry into the New York City Marathon if they run nine New York Road

Runners club races and volunteer to serve at one. Mostly though, people volunteer because they have humble servant's hearts.

My favorite Biblical servant, other than Jesus, is John the Baptist. Mark introduces him in immediately in Mark 1:1-5: "The beginning of the gospel of Jesus Christ, the Son of God, just as it is written in Isaiah the prophet: 'Behold, I am sending My messenger before You, Who will prepare Your way; The voice of one calling out in the wilderness, 'Prepare the way of the Lord, Make His paths straight!' John the Baptist appeared in the wilderness, preaching a baptism of repentance for the forgiveness of sins. And all the country of Judea was going out to him, and all the people of Jerusalem; and they were being baptized by him in the Jordan River, confessing their sins."

Two quick things we should note about John from these verses. The first is that he was the fulfillment of Isaiah's prophecy. It's no small thing to fulfill the words of God. John was the expected one who would prepare the way for Jesus. The second thing we should notice is that everyone was going out to the wilderness to see him. To many, he was a curiosity. They thought, "Let's go out and see this guy who dresses in camel hair, eats locusts, and preaches a baptism of repentance." John was different! But no matter the reason they went out to him, John was famous throughout Israel.

Fame is a very dangerous thing. It can be intoxicating. Like liquor or praise, it can go to our heads and cause us to misperceive reality. It can cause us to think more of ourselves than we should. We can get used to reading our own press clippings and develop an inflated ego and massive pride. We only need to look at famous athletes, Hollywood celebrities, and politicians to know this is true. Yet that never happened to John. His message from the very beginning was, "After me One is coming who is mightier than I, and I am not fit to bend down and untie the straps of His sandals. I baptized you with water; but He will baptize you with the Holy Spirit" (Mark 1:7-8.)

When Jesus appeared on the scene, even He asked John to baptize Him. John objected. He had baptized everyone who came out to him in the wilderness, but he knew that baptizing Jesus would be a reversal of roles. John said in Matthew 3:14: "I have the need to be baptized by You, and yet You are coming to me?" John only agreed after Jesus reassured him, saying, "Allow it at this time; for in this way it is fitting for us to fulfill all righteousness."

Later, a group came to him in John 3:26 and said to him, "Rabbi, He who was with you beyond the Jordan, to whom you have testified—behold, He is baptizing and all the people are coming to Him." John answered, "You yourselves are my witnesses that I said, 'I am not the Christ,' but, 'I have been sent ahead of Him.' He who has the bride is the groom; but the friend of the groom, who stands and listens to him, rejoices greatly because of the groom's voice. So this joy of mine has been made full. He must increase, but I must decrease." (John 3:28-30.)

What a statement of humility! It's so contrary to human nature. We're always seeking to become greater, to receive affirmation, praise, and glory from others. Deep in our hearts, we crave the praise of men. That's why Jesus warned about it in John 5:44, saying, "How can you believe, when you accept glory from one another and you do not seek the glory that is from the one and only God?"

John's statement is so shocking because it's so rare. Who would ever say, "He must increase, but I must decrease?" Only a truly humble person would say those words. Humility is not thinking less of yourself, it's thinking of yourself less. That was John's attitude. To be a humble servant of the Lord, we need to think of ourselves less. We're ready to fill any role, no matter how menial, or below our perceived station in life. Christians should understand that service is a God given opportunity to display our humility and show the world the love of Christ. We're not likely to do this on our own. We can do it by submitting to the will of God through the power of the Holy Spirit inside. As we yield to the Father's will, He makes us more like Christ.

If ever there was a humble servant, it was Jesus. He said in Mark 10:45: "For even the Son of Man did not come to be served, but to serve, and to give His life as a ransom for many." Then Jesus willingly went to the cross to pay for the sins of the very people who killed Him, and yours and mine too. What a glorious God we serve! I thank Jesus for His humble sacrifice every day.

Whenever I take a cup of water from a volunteer, I thank them if I have any breath left in my lungs! I try to throw my empty cup in a garbage can instead of on the ground to make their job easier. I also try to thank the police officers out on the course directing traffic. They keep distracted racers like me from getting run over! Simple appreciation is the least we can do for these volunteers who faithfully serve us. Whenever we have the chance, we should pay that service forward to others. God loves it when we say, "He must increase, but I must decrease."

CHAPTER 27

SHOCK WAVE THERAPY

OVER THE LAST couple of years, I've increased my mileage significantly. I'm running half-marathons frequently and training for three full marathons in the coming months. I feel great about my overall fitness, but my knees are really barking at me. In fact, during my last long run, I had to stop because of the pain. That's discouraging since I have a full marathon scheduled a month from now. I've been going to a chiropractor for the past few years to help keep me aligned and to work out kinks in my muscles. It's helped keep me on the road. A few visits ago, I told him about my aching knees, and he suggested shock wave therapy. To me, that brought back images of Jack Nicholson in "One Flew Over the Cuckoo's Nest." I wasn't interested. Then he explained that shock wave therapy treats physical pain by sending high energy acoustic waves into your hurting joints. The treatment promotes regeneration of bones, tendons, and other soft tissues.

I'm a bit of a skeptic about treatment that isn't traditional medicine or surgery, but it's non-invasive, and I figured I had nothing to lose. Off we went to the shock therapy treatment

room. He smeared gel on my knees and then took out his magic
shock wave therapy wand and started moving it over my knees,
asking me to tell him when I felt pain. Once I grimaced in pain,
he eased up the intensity of the shock waves and told me to tell
him when I reached my pain threshold. We did this for about
10 minutes on each knee. It hurt, but we could control the pain.
I asked when I might notice results. He said I might detect a
difference the next day. The next day, I went for a run, and I
was amazed. The pain wasn't gone, but it was significantly
better. I went about 5 miles in relative comfort. I tried it again
the next day. This time I went 7 miles with similar results. I'd
say I'm at least 50% better, and that's after only one treatment!

I've been thinking about the mystery and wonder of a
magic wand that can remove my pain simply by contacting my
knee in the right place at the proper setting. Modern medicine
is a marvel to me. Who knows what they will devise next? Or
who knows what medical treatments are to come? My musings
brought me to spiritual matters. One trait all human beings
share is our sin nature. We inherited it from Adam and Eve,
who sinned in the Garden of Eden. Since then, every person
has been born with a sin nature. Because of it, we all sin. Our
sin separates us from God and sets us on the road to eternity
apart from Him. We need a cure for this spiritual problem that
theologians sometimes call "the human predicament." Modern
medicine can cure lots of physical ills and help us live longer,
more productive lives, but it can't fix the human predicament.

Thankfully, Jesus came to save us from the penalty of our
sin. Because we are sinners who can do nothing to save
ourselves, and because God loves us so much, He sent Jesus to
live a sinless life and then take the punishment we deserve by
dying on a cross in our place. This didn't coincidently happen
to Jesus. He wasn't a victim of bad luck, or bad people. Before
time, the Trinity planned for this. After His death, they buried

Him in a tomb, where He remained for three days until His glorious resurrection on Easter Sunday. Jesus is alive again! Jesus proved that death had no hold over Him, and He promises us that if we believe in Him, death will not hold us either. Romans 8:11 promises: "But if the Spirit of Him who raised Jesus from the dead dwells in you, He who raised Christ Jesus from the dead will also give life to your mortal bodies through His Spirit who dwells in you."

That's an astounding promise! To know with absolute certainty that God will raise us from death to eternal life with Him, all we need is the Spirit of God living inside us. How do we get it? There's only one way. It's not by doing good works. We don't have God's Spirit living inside because we go to church or because someone baptized us. God's Spirit lives inside us when we believe in Jesus Christ alone for our salvation. We trust that though we have no power to save ourselves, because we have trusted in Jesus to save us, we possess the Holy Spirit. The Holy Spirit indwells every believer and promises us eternal life. God gives us this amazing gift that heals our human predicament like a magic wand, simply because we believe. What may seem like a magic wand to us came at infinite cost to God. He had to watch sinful, hate-filled humans kill His beloved Son to offer the gift to us. All we need to do is receive it.

I've got two runs under my belt after my first shock wave therapy treatment. So far, so good. Maybe it works, and my bones, tendons, and soft tissue have experienced some regeneration. But I'm a realist. I don't expect this to be a miracle cure. The pain could come back, and my knees may deteriorate as I run and age. I may even need knee replacement in the future. Shock wave therapy is a temporary and imperfect cure to my physical problem. Jesus is the final and perfect solution to our spiritual problem. I never have to worry that my spiritual condition will deteriorate. God has saved me. He has regenerated my soul, and nothing can ever change that. When Jesus returns, I'll get a new body with perfect knees. I'll be able to run around heaven all I want, but only because God has fixed my spiritual problem and rescued me from the human predicament. Has He fixed yours?

CHAPTER 28

ACCEPT YOURSELF?

I PICKED up my friend for lunch recently and headed toward our favorite Tex-Mex Restaurant. On the way, a Chinese Buffet caught my eye. I love a good buffet and my friend was game, so in we went. We gorged on salmon, shrimp, squid, dumplings, and some other foods I've never even heard of. Then for dessert, we ate self-serve ice cream, and various cakes, pies, and puddings. It's not exactly proper fuel for race training, but occasionally you have to go big.

As we finished lunch, along with the check, our server brought us fortune cookies. Mine said, "Always accept yourself the way you are." What's your initial reaction to that statement? I know it was intended to make me feel good about myself, to give myself grace, and not beat myself up constantly for past mistakes. Those are Christian principles. God wants us to receive His forgiveness and heal our wounds. Once we do, we shouldn't continue to carry around the guilt and shame of our sins. We leave them at the cross, accept that God will use our mistakes for good, and we get on with our lives. We also receive with joy the spiritual gifts God gives to us. It's not right to harbor jealousy over someone else's gifts. God wants us to accept the gifts He has given us with joy and use them for the glory of His kingdom. I get all that, but my initial reaction to my fortune was revulsion!

As a runner and as a Christian, I'm not ready to accept myself the way I am. On the road, I'm continually trying to run faster or longer. Every time I race, I believe I have another PR in me, and I go for it. My mindset is always, "If I could just shave one second per mile, I'll get it." Then I train with those goals in mind. As a Christian, God's not through with me yet. If He were, He'd have already taken me home to glory. Since He hasn't, I continue to seek His will, and ask Him to shape me and mold me into who He wants me to be.

Someone once said, "God loves you just the way you are, but He loves you too much to leave you that way." The first part means that God will meet each one of us right where we are at that moment. We may have committed the most heinous crimes, the most immoral acts of debauchery, or the most unethical business deals in history. But if we turn to God and ask forgiveness, and receive Jesus as our Savior, God will forgive us and give us the gift of eternal life. He loves us just as we are, and will reject no one who comes to Him, no matter what we've done. But God's not done with us. The second part of that statement is He loves us too much to leave us in our wretched, sinful state. He wants us to change our behavior and make us less selfish, so we'll live for Him and for others.

These commands to change are all over the Bible. For example, Colossians 3:5 says: "Put to death, therefore, whatever belongs to your earthly nature: sexual immorality, impurity, lust, evil desires and greed, which is idolatry." Galatians 2:20 says: "I have been crucified with Christ and I no longer live, but Christ lives in me. The life I now live in the body, I live by faith in the Son of God, who loved me and gave himself for me." Romans 6:6-7 says: "Our old self was crucified with Him, in order that our body of sin might be done away with, so that we would no longer be slaves to sin; for the one who has died is freed from sin."

The theological word for becoming more like Jesus is "sanctification." It means, "to set aside as holy," or "to purify." That's what God wants for us after He's saved us. God doesn't just blindly hope that we'll become more like Jesus, He gives us the means to do it and guides the process. When God saved us, He gave us His Holy Spirit, the third person of the Trinity, God Himself, to live inside us. Romans 8:9 says: "But if anyone does not have the Spirit of Christ, he does not belong to Him." One ministry of the Holy Spirit is to make us more like Christ. God saved us in our state of reprehensible sin, but now that He has saved us, He wants to clean up our lives. That means killing sin wherever the Holy Spirit reveals it to us, and obeying God's moral and ethical laws so we look more like Jesus. This doesn't happen overnight. It's a lifelong process, which is why I objected to my fortune cookie. Just like I want to run faster every time I race, I want to become more like Jesus every day.

The more I thought about my fortune, the more I realized that the source of my disagreement with it is the word "always." As I've said, I'm 56 now. Statistics say that I'm on the backside of the hill and that my best physical fitness is behind me. I accept that I won't run a PR every time out, and that aches and pains will slow me down. But the word "always" implies resignation and hopelessness to me. It means that I should give up and not keep trying to improve even as I age. I'm just not ready for that.

In my Christian walk, to "always" accept myself the way I am means to become complacent, resting on my laurels, and satisfied with my station on the journey. Once I adopt that mindset, I'm finished growing. God doesn't want us to become spiritual "fat cats." He wants people who are useful to Him in building His kingdom. Spiritual growth only happens as we acknowledge daily that we are not who God wants us to be. We wake up every morning asking God to teach us something new today. God constantly presents us with opportunities to serve Him and His people if we're willing to pay attention. He'll ask us to serve in ways that might make us uncomfortable. We rely on God's power to do His will through us.

In the movie, *Annie Hall*, Woody Allen's character says to his girlfriend played by Diane Keaton, "A relationship, I think, is like a shark, you know? It has to constantly move forward, or it dies. And I think what we got on our hands here is a dead shark." That's brilliant, and it sums up my feelings about running and my walk with the Lord. I'm not ready to stop moving forward and die. Accept myself the way I am? In certain situations. "Always" accept myself the way I am? Never!

CHAPTER 29

I FELT LIKE I WAS GOING TO DIE

ALL RUNNERS HAVE THOUGHT they might die during a run! For some reason, our bodies won't cooperate. Maybe it's a random pain, or bad tacos the night before. We'd planned a run of x miles, and we can't even make half of it. I had a run like that recently. I aimed for 20 miles as part of my marathon training program. My knees were killing me, so I compensated by changing my stride, leaning forward as I ran to relieve the pressure. That didn't work. My form suffered, and my heart rate escalated to an unsustainable level. I made it 15 miles and had to stop. In short, I felt like I was going to die! Doesn't this make you want to run right now?

I listen to a lot of podcasts when I run. My Facebook running group recommended the "Freakonomics" Podcast. During this run, I was listening to an episode where the host interviewed Dr. B.J. Miller on death and dying. Not exactly an uplifter, especially when I felt like this topic might be extremely relevant in the next few minutes! Dr. Miller argued that our model of dying is all wrong. Instead of submitting to every kind of treatment imaginable in hospitals to extend our lives for a few more minutes, hours, days, or months, we should weigh the quantity of our lives against the quality of our lives. There's a better way to die, and that's by accepting death as a natural part of life. When death is inevitable, we ought to embrace it and use the time to reconcile with people, tell people how much we love them, and otherwise prepare.

I respect Dr. Miller's opinion and agree with it, but not for the reasons he said. Neither Dr. Miller, nor the host, mentioned God in the entire podcast. Two main reasons people resist death are surely their fear of pain or discomfort during dying, but more importantly, their uncertainty of what comes next. We have a medical doctor in our church who also doubles as his hospital's bioethics chairperson. I have listened to him teach several times about the ethical issues surrounding death and dying, answering questions like, when should doctors encourage people to stop receiving medical treatment, and if the sick cannot decide for themselves, when should the family stop medical intervention and allow natural processes to run their course?

He said in his experience, the single most important factor for the dying person or for their families in making these hard decisions is whether those dying know they are going to heaven. No one wants to endure the process of death, but for those who long to see Jesus and know they will, death is just a gateway to the heavenly home Jesus promised. It's a lot easier to surrender this life when you have peace about what's next. The podcast didn't even touch this most important issue. How can anyone have peace of mind in death, or release their lives a minute earlier than possible if they're unsure of what's next? Or if they believe this life is all there is and then nothingness?

I can only concentrate on a podcast for the first hour of a run. After that, my brain turns to mush, and I switch to music and just let my mind roam around. One song on my playlist is

"Like a Stone" by Audioslave. I love the song but had never considered the lyrics before. Chris Cornell was the lead singer of Audioslave. I don't know if he wrote the lyrics, but his haunting voice sings of despair and desperation. He's seeking a way into heaven after a life of regret, but not knowing how to get there. He anticipates lying on his deathbed praying to gods and angels like a pagan praying to anyone who would take him to heaven. They describe a man who longs to be in God's house, but waits for death unsure, alone, lifeless, like a stone. Chris Cornell died by suicide in 2017. I don't know if he ever received Jesus as his Savior and is now enjoying the peace, forgiveness, and rest in God's house he longed for in life.

Today, October 1, is our 28th wedding anniversary. I don't want to think about life without Molly, but inevitably, one of us will predecease the other. Death is a most unpleasant concept for those without faith in Jesus and His promises. Few people want to talk about it, but we all will experience it. A wiser approach would be to accept death's reality and plan for it now. We prepare by making peace with God. The only way to have peace with God is to accept Jesus as our Savior from our sins. Romans 5:8-10 says: "But God demonstrates His own love toward us, in that while we were still sinners, Christ died for us. Much more then, having now been justified by His blood, we shall be saved from the wrath of God through Him. For if while we were enemies we were reconciled to God through the death of His Son, much more, having been reconciled, we shall be saved by His life."

These verses beautifully encapsulate the gospel. They show us why we don't need to fear death. Our sin once sepa-rated us from God, but through Jesus' death for us, we have peace with God if we have believed in Jesus as our Savior. Jesus took on our sin and gave us His righteousness. Christians don't fear death because Jesus paid the price for our sin and reconciled us to God. We won't face the wrath we deserve for our sin. Instead, He will welcome us into His kingdom.

We're all philosophers on some level. Philosophy means "love of wisdom." Philosophers try to understand truths about themselves, the world, their relationships, the meaning of their existence, and what happens when we die. Dr. Miller and Chris Cornell philosophized about death and dying. In their musings though, they both left out the most important detail. Chris Cornell's journey has ended, while Dr. Miller's and countless others' lives continue during their time on earth. As Christians, we should pray they find the only source of peace in dying. We should look for opportunities to share our faith with those who don't yet believe.

On my run, I may have felt like I was going to die. I've felt like that many times and haven't died yet! In a few minutes, I got my breath back and recovered. It disappointed me that I couldn't make the entire 20 miles I had planned. I also knew that 15 miles is better than none, and I'll try again next week. Someday though, I'll have to face the reality of dying. I'll probably fear the dying process. No one wants pain and suffering. But I'll have no fear or anxiety about where I'm going. I've already got that settled with God. Because of that, I hope I'll take Dr. Miller's advice to let my life go, rather than prolong it unnecessarily. I know Jesus is waiting for me on the other side.

CHAPTER 30

FEAR OF PAIN

MY LONG TRAINING run last week wasn't pleasant. I could summarize it in one word: pain. My knees, feet, and shoulders hurt, and even my lungs were gasping for breath at the end. Training for a long race takes months. It would be amazing if we could be "marathon ready" after one long run. Unfortunately, when training for a marathon, the long run comes every week. Like waves on the beach, the long run is relentless in its coming. We've barely recovered from last week before we have to do it again this week. Considering last week's long run causes me to fear this week's.

I'm thinking about changes I could make before Saturday to improve my run. I resolved to drink more water during the week, not just the day before the run. The new shoes I bought just arrived in the mail. I went to the chiropractor for an adjustment. I started taking Turmeric and Collagen II for my joints and bones. Borrowing from Forrest Gump, "Running is like a box of chocolates. You never know what you're gonna get." Every run is different and unpredictable. Saturday morning is coming fast. If I want to be marathon ready, I have to hit the road again and properly prepare to have a better day than last week. And pray!

Jesus always knew what He was going to get. He told His disciples three times in Mark's gospel that He was going up to Jerusalem, where the religious leaders would mock Him, spit on Him, abuse Him, and kill Him. The disciples couldn't understand how their Messiah could die. Peter chastised Jesus for making these predictions. Jesus responded to Peter in Matthew 16:23: "Get behind Me, Satan! You are a stumbling block to Me; for you are not setting your mind on God's purposes, but men's." Jesus never wavered from His mission. Luke 9:51 says, "When the days were approaching for His ascension, He was determined to go to Jerusalem." His determination to go to Jerusalem to suffer and die is astounding to me. It is way beyond the fear of the next long run!

In the Garden of Gethsemane, Jesus asked the Father if there was another way to accomplish the salvation of humanity so He wouldn't have to go to the cross. In Luke 22:42, Jesus said to God, "Father, if You are willing, remove this cup from Me; yet not My will, but Yours be done." This was Jesus showing his full humanity, not wanting the pain of the cross. God didn't remove the cup of suffering from Jesus. Instead, He sent angels to strengthen Him for the task at hand. Luke 22:44-45: "And being in agony, He was praying very fervently; and His sweat became like drops of blood, falling down upon the ground. Jesus said to God, 'Not my will Father, but yours.'"

Within the hour, the Roman soldiers arrested Jesus and brought Him to the Jewish leaders. They convicted Him of heresy and sentenced Him to death, but Jewish law prevented them from executing Jesus. Only Romans could employ capital punishment. The Jews brought Him to Pilate and charged Jesus with heresy for claiming to be God. Pilate was a Roman pagan. He didn't care if Jesus blasphemed the Jewish God. The

Jewish leaders then changed the charge against Jesus to sedition, saying that Jesus called Himself a king. That got Pilate's attention. A rival king was a challenge to Rome, and Pilate had to take that seriously. After questioning Jesus, he found no reason to execute Him. Pilate didn't want to crucify Jesus. He hoped that a good flogging would satisfy the crowd.

The beating Jesus received would have killed many men. The Romans used a cord of leather strips embedded with bone fragments and pieces of metal to whip their victims. This whip would have dug into Jesus' flesh and ripped chunks of it right off His back. The Jews limited flogging to 39 lashes, but the Romans had no restrictions. They could continue to their heart's content. We don't know how many lashes Jesus received. After it was over, Pilate brought Him out to the crowd and said, "Behold the man." Jesus' bloodthirsty enemies only cried out louder for Pilate to crucify Jesus.

When Pilate could find no politically safe way to release Jesus, he handed Him over for crucifixion. Jesus hung on a cross for six hours before He died. Jesus suffered excruciating physical pain, but also the loss of fellowship with His Father for the only time in eternity. No man ever suffered as Jesus did. The amazing thing is that Jesus knew this day was coming, and still He walked ahead of the crowd, setting His face toward Jerusalem, knowing what awaited Him there. Talk about fear of pain! Can you imagine knowing the agonizing suffering and death that awaited you?

Somehow, even with His death in view, Jesus lived a joyful life. He laughed, loved, and lived with His friends, not allowing the future suffering on the cross to ruin the joy of each day. He could focus on the glory He would receive after He did the work God sent Him to do.

That's a bit like how I approach the long run. I know it's coming, but I'm willing to endure it for the glory of finishing a marathon. When the long run comes, I pray that my body will hold up and that I can complete whatever goal I've set. I fear the pain, but if I can just get through that day's run, I'll be better prepared for the big race ahead. It's a sacrifice I'm willing to make.

Runners use the phrase, "no pain, no gain," to say we're willing to endure the pain of running to improve fitness. During the long training run, we're willing to tolerate certain thresholds of agony as an investment in our goals. For Jesus, "no pain, no gain," meant if He didn't go to the cross to suffer for us, He could not have saved humanity from the penalty of sin. The next time we're running our long run, or any time we experience the suffering of life, we should remember the excruciating pain Jesus endured for us. It's a great way to take the focus off our own pain and help us praise the Savior.

CHAPTER 31

SECOND CHANCES

I REALLY MISS the beach since we moved to Texas. When we lived in New Jersey, I took day trips to the beach for granted. Now, whenever I visit my parents in Florida, I always I go to the ocean. I love the smell of the beach, feeling the sand under my feet, and hearing the waves crash. Seeing the beauty of God's creation draws me closer to Him and brings me peace.

I haven't run on the beach in years, and since I'm trying to prevent injury before a big race coming up in a couple of weeks, I walked instead. God created the Sabbath so we would rest, and runners need rest too! As I walked the beach, I saw several people casting fishing lines into the surf. I rarely see anyone catch a fish, but this time one of them had a fish on. I stopped to watch. You never know what's going to be on the other end of the line. He reeled it in and pulled it out of the water. I'm not sure what kind of fish it was, but it wasn't even a foot long. He looked at it with disdain and disappointment, pulled the hook out of its mouth and tossed it back. Experience gained and a second chance for that lucky fish.

. . .

If that fish had been a little bigger, there would have been no second chance. That fish would have been on his plate that night. As I walked on, I thought about how God continually gives us second chances and how we learn by knowledge and experience how to live His way. Imagine ourselves as the fish and the bait as temptation to sin. Every metaphor breaks down eventually. Who is the fisher in mine? To help my metaphor work, let's imagine Satan as the fisher baiting the hook and casting it in the water, but God as the fisher when He releases the fish. (True, the fisher wouldn't have released a bigger fish, but work with me here!)

Satan casts the bait. It looks so good, and we think it will give us pleasure, or improve our lives. That's the nature of temptation. Satan uses it like he used the forbidden fruit with Eve, to make her think she was missing out on the good stuff, and that her life wouldn't be complete without it. He made Eve want the fruit so badly that she ate. Satan uses different bait to catch different fish. He knows what tempts you and what tempts me. The bait could be sexual sin, desire for riches, pride in our achievements, or many sins that look so good. We only realize sin's hook has snagged us after we've swallowed the bait. Once we're caught, the devil wants to hold us there, enslaved to sin and its consequences and never able to get off the hook.

God wants us to be free from sin, not only from its penalty, but also from its power. Faith in Jesus saves us from the penalty of sin. Dependence on the indwelling Holy Spirit saves us from the power of sin. Paul wrote in Romans 6:11-12: "Even so consider yourselves to be dead to sin, but alive to God in Christ Jesus. Therefore, do not let sin reign in your mortal body so that you obey its lusts." To be dead to sin means that we no longer allow it to hold its power over us. Sin cannot entice dead things. When presented with the opportunity to sin, we consider ourselves dead regarding the bait of sin so it cannot ensnare us. While we consider ourselves dead to sin, we remember that we're alive to Christ, so we should seek God's desires for us.

1 Corinthians 10:13 says, "No temptation has overtaken you but such as is common to man; and God is faithful, who will not allow you to be tempted beyond what you are able, but with the temptation will provide the way of escape also, so that you will be able to endure it." The way of escape in 1 Corinthians 10:13 is to consider ourselves dead to sin but alive to God in Christ Jesus. Let's be real though. None of us can do this every time we encounter temptation. That's why we need a Savior! As we grow as Christians, we'll gain more experience. Like a fish will only grow to adulthood by recognizing and avoiding danger, we'll only grow in Christ by recognizing Satan's bait and ignoring it. It looks enticing and may satisfy in the short term, but it often leads to extremely painful and unwanted consequences, even death.

Continuing the metaphor, think about the grace of God. How many times has Satan caught us on the hook of temptation and wouldn't let us go? He would hold us forever if he could, but God took the hook from our big, fat, lustful, greedy mouths, gave us another chance, and threw us back into the ocean. A little bloodied and beaten up but still alive with wisdom gained. It's only because of God's love and grace that He can do that. By all rights, we should end up filleted, cooked, and served. But our God of love and grace doesn't want that for us. Instead, He says to us as Jesus said to the woman caught in adultery, "I do not condemn you, either. Go. From now on sin no more" (John 8:11.)

God doesn't just release us from sin only once. He does it repeatedly. He forgives, and forgives, and forgives those who repent. That doesn't mean that He won't allow us to suffer consequences of our sin, but He doesn't make us pay the penalty we deserve, which is eternal separation from Him in hell. Jesus didn't come to catch us *in* sin, but to save us *from* it. He's the great God of second chances and new life. May we receive the gift and live worthy of it.

CHAPTER 32

MY BEST FAN

LIKE MOST OF you who are training for a race or maintaining your current level of fitness, the Saturday morning long run is a staple in my life. For me, that usually means 10 miles or more. I run a three-mile loop that brings me back to the house where I stash water and snacks to keep me going. My favorite part of the long run is knowing that there will probably be a short little encouraging note on an index card waiting for me after every loop. They're from my wife Molly, by best fan. Last Saturday, she left four separate notes. The first one said, "I'm proud of you!" On the second, she wrote, "You can do it!" The third one said, "Shut up knees, you're fine!" That one cracked me up. A last one said, "You can do it! No bad attitudes!" It was perfect for how I was feeling at that very moment.

She supports me not only on the Saturday long run, but she comes to every race. She looks at the course map, plans how she can see me the most times on the course, and tells me where she will be. Runners love when fans cheer them on, but it's extra special when that fan is the one you love more than anyone else and who loves you the same way. If she says I'll see you at the 7-mile mark, I run the entire 7th mile waiting to see her. What an emotional boost I get knowing she will be there with a smile, a high-five, and a cheer of encouragement. The adrenaline of seeing her will sustain me for the 8th mile too. Then I can begin counting down until the next place she will station herself.

Runners will use anything for a psychological boost. Knowing I'll see her every few miles helps me break a long race down into manageable segments. When the running is hard, I tell myself it's only two miles until I see her again. These bits of encouragement sustain me. Though she's not running side by side with me, I feel her presence with me every step of the way.

Running is self-inflicted madness. We can stop whenever we want. Unfortunately, the pain of life isn't like that. We don't have the power to turn it off when it seems unbearable. Fortunately for Christians, we have Jesus, walking beside us every step of the way, enduring our pain and guilt with us, and encouraging us to lean on Him when life seems too much to bear.

In Matthew 11: 28-30, Jesus said, "Come to me, all you who are weary and burdened, and I will give you rest. Take my yoke upon you and learn from me, for I am gentle and humble in heart, and you will find rest for your souls. For my yoke is easy and my burden is light." In context, Jesus was combating the teaching of the scribes and Pharisees, who added burdens and conditions to the law of Moses and stood aloof over the people, judging them harshly. They added to the load rather than lightening it. A yoke was a wooden frame that joined two oxen together to plow a field or pull a load. The yoke that the scribes and Pharisees placed on the people was too much to bear. Jesus did not say, "Come to my teaching, my philosophy, or my law." He said, "Come to Me."

. . .

The scribes and Pharisees believed in salvation through strict adherence to rules and regulations that no one, not even they, could keep. Jesus invites us to lay down the burdens of the law as a way of salvation, and simply come to Him. Jesus invites us to release ourselves from the weight of all the guilt and shame we carry. All the sin we've ever committed, Jesus takes on Himself so we can have rest while we live. For burdened souls, Jesus is the source and the place of rest, peace, and comfort for our souls. He frees us from the yoke.

In John Bunyan's, *The Pilgrim's Progress*, the great allegory of Christian salvation, the main character "Christian" carried a load on his back until He climbed a hill with a cross at the top. At the cross, the burden fell off Christian's shoulders. God took it from him and freed him to continue his journey to the "Celestial Gate," (a metaphor for heaven) without it. That's what Jesus has done for us. He saved us with His work at the cross, then He walks side-by-side with us every day no matter what we're going through until we reach the Celestial Gate. Jesus is the way to salvation and our peace and comfort as we go through life. When we come to Him, He says to us, "Unburden yourself from the weight of all the guilt and shame you carry. Give me the burden of your sins and failures. Welcome to My Family! Now go live joyfully knowing that you'll never have to carry this load again. I've got it." When Christian unburdened himself at the cross, he said with a merry heart, "He has given me rest by his sorrow, and life by his death."[1] Then He continued His journey.

Molly is my best earthly fan. Not just in my running, but in my preaching, pastoring, parenting, and everything I do. I hope I am her biggest encourager too! But we can't be with each other every minute of every day. Even if we could, we're just humans. Only God can take away the shame and guilt of our sins. Jesus is our biggest fan. No matter what we've done, He's always by our side. He never rejects us, but takes our sin off our backs, puts it on His own and encourages us on our journey. Like Molly's notes, Jesus says, "I'm proud of you!" "You can do it. No bad attitudes!"

When life is hard and the burden seems too great to bear, don't carry it yourself. Give it to Jesus. He will carry it for you and run alongside you. He'll be your biggest fan, cheering you on to the finish line.

CHAPTER 33

UNFRIENDLY RUNNERS

BECAUSE I RUN the same routes, I see familiar faces on almost every run. Most runners are eager to wave and say hello. We're members of a common fraternity of crazy people who understand each other. I love waving to other runners and am shocked when other runners don't wave back! Almost every Saturday morning, I see a couple of runners who I presume are mother and daughter. I don't know how many times I have passed them on the road, but they have never once returned my wave. How rude! Do I have a glop of mayonnaise on my face or something? I can't figure it out. I have two options. Should I just ignore them and stop waving, or should I wave more enthusiastically to elicit a response. What to do?

I'm not the most extroverted guy in the world, but I try to be friendly. I don't think anyone would describe me as a troublesome person. Even so, I have difficult people in my life as I'm sure you do too. There are some people who we just can't seem to get along with. Our personalities don't mesh. We get under each other's skin. In those circumstances, we can try even harder, or we can choose to avoid those people. This translates to evangelism too. It's hard in the best circumstances to talk to an unbeliever about Jesus. But when the person we're trying to talk to seems hardened to the gospel and anything related to God, it feels like a waste of time. Even Jesus recognized this as a problem. He said in the Sermon on the Mount, "Do not give what is holy to dogs, and do not throw your pearls before swine, or they will trample them under their feet, and turn and tear you to pieces" (Matthew 7:6.)

Jesus seems very harsh in these verses, calling people dogs and swine. What did He mean? The pearls and what is holy are references to the gospel. The swine and the dogs were the people who were unreceptive to it. Swine and dogs were unclean animals in the Old Testament. If one touched a dog or swine, it made them ceremonially unclean and they couldn't worship in the temple (Leviticus 11:7.) Peter heard the Sermon on the Mount in person. Thirty years later, he wrote about false prophets, slaves of depravity, and anyone else hostile to the Kingdom of God, calling them dogs and swine. In 2 Peter 2:22, he wrote, "Of them the proverbs are true, 'A dog returns to its vomit,' and, 'A sow that is washed returns to her wallowing in the mud.'" Paul said in Philippians 2:3, "Beware of the dogs; beware of the evildoers; beware of the false circumcision." Dogs and swine are not mere unbelievers. God always expects us to witness to unbelievers. Dogs and swine are those so hardened and hostile that God excuses us from speaking to them, to throwing what is holy to them. Even Jesus refused to speak to Herod in Luke 23:9. He knew Herod wouldn't believe.

How will we know who is too hostile to hear the gospel? Only by trying to share it with them. If they prove to be so hostile that continuing to try with them is a waste of time, start praying for them rather than talking to them. Salvation is God's work. He can change their hearts. Most times we don't share the gospel because it's too much effort. We're afraid of rejection, or we fear we don't have all the answers to the questions they'll ask, and we don't want to be embarrassed. It's rare that we don't share the gospel because people are hostile. Most evangelists say they almost never receive hostility or ridicule. Our obligation is to share the truth about Jesus and leave the results to Him.

Sometimes we should withhold the gospel, when by the power of the Holy Spirit, we discern the person too hostile to receive the good news. That should be the very rare exception rather than the rule. God is in the business of changing hearts and saving souls. There's no one beyond His reach. If we judge that someone is too hostile to receive the gospel after many attempts, we should grieve for that person and pray for them.

Now back to these two ladies that I so frequently pass on my Saturday long runs. I'm not calling them dogs or swine! My question is, is it worth it to keep waving to them every Saturday morning even though they continue to rebuff my friendly greeting? I think it is. Persistence pays. It's true in running. We get in better shape as we continue to hit the road day after day. Persistence pays in relationships too. We build better relationships by being together and working out conflict. Persistence pays in anything we do. It also pays in evangelism. Persistent prayer and sharing the gospel makes disciples. So being the persistent fellow I am, I will continue to wave to these ladies. One Saturday morning I will have my reward when they shock me by waving back!

P.S. I saw the daughter on my long run this morning. I stepped up my wave game big time, fully raising my left arm over my shoulder and shouting a heart-felt, "Good Morning!" Crickets. Not even a little eye contact! I'll try again next week!

CHAPTER 34

A STRONG CORE

ARTICLES ABOUT RUNNING FILL my email inbox every day. Recently I read one about how important it is to have a strong core. The body's core includes the chest, back, abs and obliques. Increased core strength stabilizes the torso, improves balance, provides a solid foundation for the body, and improves posture and speed. On long runs or races, when we're fatigued, our form suffers. Having a strong core helps keep us balanced and able to finish strong. Those are a bunch of noble reasons to have a strong core, but the work involved! Planks, superman, windshield wipers, crunches, burpees; the words alone are enough to make me shudder. The one thing these exercises have in common is pain! If we do them consistently, we'll develop a strong core, but did I mention the pain?!

I have attempted core exercises over the years. In my forties, I consistently did some of these workouts for almost a year. Truthfully, I'd rather run 10 miles than do 15 minutes of core work. That's how much I hate strengthening my abs. So mostly, I've ignored my core. Doctors and physiologists say that I'll pay the price for that in the future, and I'm sure they're right. I can still run long distances and log about 25-30 miles weekly, but I have a little jelly in the belly, and I already suffer minor aches and pains that I'm sure a strong core would help. Maybe someday (sigh.)

One place where I try to maintain a strong core is in my faith. As any Christian knows, there are many, many, denominations of Christianity. At the highest level, Christians divide between Catholics, Protestants, and Eastern Orthodox. Within Protestantism and Eastern Orthodoxy, there are hundreds, if not thousands, of denominations. There are even different denominations within Catholicism. Sometimes the distinguishing features between denominations are minor points of theology, sometimes the points are major. How do we know the difference? By having a strong core. We must understand the non-negotiables of the Christian faith. We could call these cardinal doctrines of the faith, without which we would no longer have Christianity. Examples of these are Jesus' birth by the virgin Mary, Jesus' deity, Jesus' death on the cross for our sin and salvation through faith in Him alone, Jesus' bodily resurrection, Jesus' second coming, and The Trinity. I don't have space here for a detailed explanation of each, but take any of them away and you no longer have Christianity.

Once we know these, it should be easy to recognize other beliefs that are not core, but which some Christians strongly hold. I would call these gray issues, or debatable areas. A gray issue would be one that God does not directly address in the Bible, or an issue where reasonable and faithful Christians could disagree about interpretation. Examples of gray issues include which version of the Bible is best, (King James, New International, New American, etc.) What style of worship music is appropriate? (Hymns vs. worship music; Guitars and drums vs. organ and piano vs. no instruments.) Should Christians celebrate Halloween, dance, drink alcohol in moderation, or see Harry Potter movies? Should we celebrate the Lord's Supper every Sunday, every month, four times a year? What color should our new carpets be?! The list could go on and on. I'm sure many of you have either experienced church splits or at least had heated arguments over these gray issues in your own church.

I said it should be easy once we know our core beliefs to distinguish them from the gray areas. However, not everyone is well-versed in the core beliefs. One of the bigger problems in our churches is that we elevate gray issues to core beliefs, and then divide over these issues about which God has not clearly spoken, or which leave room for reasonable people to hold different opinions. When the Eastern Orthodox Church split from Catholic Church in 1054, some issues that caused the split were whether the Holy Spirit proceeded from the Father and the Son, or only from the Father, and whether they should use leavened or unleavened bread for Communion. The first is a secondary point of theology. The second is a matter of worship practice. These make for interesting debates, but neither is a core belief of Christianity.

It's very important that we have a strong core in our Christian faith. If we do, we'll know when it's necessary to fight about a point of doctrine or theology, or when we should just accept another's beliefs. Sometimes we should recognize that though we don't agree with them, we can have different beliefs on that issue and still be brothers and sisters in Christ. One example of such a doctrine is the second coming of Jesus Christ. Not *whether* He's coming (that's a core doctrine), but how He's coming and when He's coming. These may seem like minor points, but churches have spilt over them. Issues like, will there be a rapture of the church? Will the church go through the tribulation? Will there be a literal 1000-year kingdom on earth? If you aren't aware of these debates, don't fret. Just be aware that many Christians divide over their stances on such nuances of theology.

As Christians, we are to accept the beliefs of our brothers and sisters in Christ. Romans 14:1-4: "Accept the one whose faith is weak, without quarreling over disputable matters. One person's faith allows them to eat anything, but another, whose faith is weak, eats only vegetables. The one who eats everything must not treat with contempt the one who does not, and the one who does not eat everything must not judge the one who does, for God has accepted them. Who are you to judge someone else's servant?"

Develop a strong core. Know the difference between cardinal and gray doctrines. Accept those with whom you disagree if it's not a cardinal doctrine. I'm always amazed when I run in a race at the different sizes and shapes of runners. There are tall ones and short ones. Some are young, others are old. Some have perfect bodies, others not so much. Yet there we all are in the same race. Most of us will cross the finish line. Not all at the same time, but we'll finish. Let that be a metaphor for our faith. Though we're not all the same, all those with a strong core, who hold to the cardinal doctrines of the Christian faith, will cross the finish line into heaven.

CHAPTER 35

BECOMING A RUNNER

I DON'T KNOW when it happened, but at some point, I transitioned from someone who runs, into a runner. Can you relate to that? The difference is subtle. I used to go for a run now and then to stay in shape, or out of guilt because I ate two cheeseburgers the night before. Running wasn't something I took seriously. In my 20s and 30s, I ran about one marathon every year. I only planned my days or weekends around running if I had one coming up. I would train for about three months, but after I ran it, I stopped training and allowed myself to get out of shape again. For most of my life, I was what you might call a casual runner.

Over the past couple years, I've become much more serious about running, some might say obsessed. I don't know what's changed. Maybe it's the pandemic and the lockdowns it brought that made me appreciate being outside. It could be recognizing that I'm aging and I'm not as invincible as I once thought I was. Maybe it's knowing that if I want this body to be useful for God's Kingdom into my 70s and 80s, I need to do a better job taking care of it now. Whatever the reason, I've become a runner, rather than someone who runs.

I'm what you might call an "all or nothing" person. I'm 100% in or I'm out. There's not much middle ground with me. When I decided I was a runner, I set a goal to join a club called Half-Fanatics. To become a member, I had to complete either two half marathons in 16 days or three half marathons in 90 days. I completed three in 90 days and joined the club at the entry level, called "Neptune." Once I was in, I wanted to "level up." That means progressing through the planets based on other insane amounts of half marathons completed. I ran three half marathons in 16 days to attain Uranus level. I ran over twelve half marathons in twelve months to reach Saturn level. Then I ran two half marathons in two days to reach Jupiter level. That's where I am now. To reach Mars, I need to complete three half marathons in three days, or over 26 in one year, or four in nine days. I don't know if I'll ever reach Mars, but I set a new goal for 2022. Three marathons in 90 days, and now I'm a Marathon Maniac! I can level up in that club too by running more marathons! For as long as my body will allow, I'm a runner!

I think most Christians would like to say that they are not just Christians, but Christ-followers. Another word for a Christ-follower is a disciple. It's really easy to become a Christian. All we need to do is to admit we're sinners who can't save ourselves and put our faith in Jesus Christ alone for salvation. When we do that, we're Christians. God saves us from punishment for our sin and gives us eternal life in Heaven. But God doesn't want casual Christians. If we truly are Christians, we should not be so in name only. The Holy Spirit should transform us into committed Christ followers who are continually seeking to sin less and grow in our faith. Jesus said in Matthew 16:24-25: "If anyone wants to come after Me, he must deny himself, take up his cross, and follow Me. For whoever wants to save his life will lose it; but whoever loses his life for My sake will find it." Like transforming from someone who runs to a runner requires commitment and cost, so does becoming a true disciple of Jesus. A true disciple of Christ is 100% in, come what may.

Jesus said in Luke 14:27-30: "Whoever does not carry his own cross and come after Me cannot be My disciple. For which one of you, when he wants to build a tower, does not first sit down and calculate the cost, to see if he has enough to complete it? Otherwise, when he has laid a foundation and is not able to finish, all who are watching it will begin to ridicule him, saying, 'This person began to build, and was not able to finish!'" The cost of discipleship is great, but if we are going to become all God wants us to become, to move from a casual Christian to a committed disciple, we must pay the cost.

What is the cost? It may be the loss of relationships, even family or friendships. It could be discrimination or ridicule at our jobs or even loss of employment. Being a disciple will most likely require us to change our lifestyle. In other countries, being a Christian may cost people their freedom and even their lives. I wonder how long it will be until Christians in America face these same challenges. The cost is high, but the rewards are great. The Christian life is a life of joy. Christians enjoy the incomparable feeling of knowing that God has forgiven our sins, and that we'll be in Heaven with our Lord and Savior forever. But that's just the beginning. When Jesus said, "Whoever loses his life for my sake will find it," He was talking about a life of joyful sacrifice of one's own life in service to others. If you've ever helped someone or given to someone in need, you know it cost you time, money, or both. But the reward is knowing that you are loving Jesus' people as He loves them. We're doing what we can to show Christ's love on earth.

Jesus said in Matthew 25:40: "Whatever you did for one of the least of these brothers and sisters of mine, you did for me." God doesn't have performance requirements to get into heaven like these running clubs. That would make salvation based on our good deeds. But God promises us rewards for service to Him. In Mark 9:41, Jesus said: "Truly I tell you, anyone who gives you a cup of water in my name because you belong to the Messiah will certainly not lose their reward."

Runners run for rewards: Health, fitness, medals, accolades, club membership, you name it. We all have our reasons for running. Whatever rewards we receive on earth will perish, but the rewards Jesus gives us are eternal. Let's not be Christians in name only. Let's commit ourselves to being disciples. A disciple is 100% in, almost obsessed with becoming more like Christ, serving His people, and making other committed disciples.

CHAPTER 36

TOOLS IN YOUR TOOLBOX

OVER THE YEARS, I've learned that I have tools in my toolbox to help me run better that I didn't know I had. For example, the toenails on my big toes are usually some shade of purple or black, and in various stages of falling off and growing back in. It's the price of being a distance runner. I'm sorry for that visual for those of you grossed out by feet. I asked for advice about this on my Facebook runners' group and received an unexpected education. Did you know that there are at least nine different ways to lace up your sneakers? I had no idea that every one of those eyelets in my running shoes has a purpose! I've been tying my shoes the same way since I was four! Now I know there's a way to tie your shoes if you have high arches, or if your heel slips in your shoes, or if you have a wide forefoot, a high arch, if your shoes feel too tight, if you have black toenails and toe pain, narrow feet, or wide feet. Who knew! Since I've been lacing my shoes to prevent "Black toe," I have noticed a difference. You should Google it!

Francis Bacon was an English philosopher and statesman who lived in the 16th century. A famous quote attributed to him is, "Knowledge is power." Time has borne out the truth of that statement. We would not have the power to cure disease without understanding its underlying cause. Infections that used to kill people are now easily curable with antibiotics because we have discovered and studied bacteria. We can fly airplanes across the world and rockets to the moon by understanding math and physics. Technology that was unknown fifty years ago powers the cell phones we can't put down today.

On the other hand, you don't know what you don't know. If I hadn't asked about black toes, I wouldn't have received valuable advice. The same is true for other aspects of running too. When I was young, I used to put my sneakers on and run without thinking about rest, nutrition, hydration, or clothing. I could get away with that in my teens and twenties. Now I know that each of these factors affects my performance and recovery. I've experimented with different drinks, gels, shorts, and shirts, and now I have a better idea of what works for me. We'll have more success if we know the tools we have and how to use them. To be a better runner, I agree with Bacon that knowledge is power.

The same principle is also true in our spiritual walk. We have tools in our spiritual toolbox to help us withstand Satan's attacks. In Ephesians 6, Paul warned that the struggles we face may appear to be against other people and the condition of the world, but the underlying cause of those struggles is spiritual. Ephesians 6:11: "For our struggle is not against flesh and blood, but against the rulers, against the powers, against the world forces of this darkness, against the spiritual forces of wickedness in the heavenly places." Paul was referring to Satan and his demons. They are behind the strife in the world.

Can you see how fighting against the wrong enemy using ineffective tools could lead to disastrous results? Paul wanted us to know who our real enemy is, so we would use the proper tools in our toolbox to defeat him. Paul identified six tools, using the metaphor of a soldier's battle gear, that we possess which will help us defeat our enemy. In Ephesians 6:13-17, Paul wrote, "Therefore, take up the full armor of God, so that you will be able to resist on the evil day, and having done everything, to stand firm. Stand firm therefore, having belted your waist with truth, and having put on the breastplate of righteousness, and having strapped on your feet the preparation of the gospel of peace; in addition to all, taking up the shield of faith with which you will be able to extinguish all the flaming arrows of the evil one. And take the helmet of salvation and the sword of the Spirit, which is the word of God."

The full armor consists of these six tools in our toolbox that God has given us to defeat Satan's attacks. 1) the belt of truth; 2) the breastplate of righteousness; 3) the gospel of peace, 4) the shield of faith; 5) the helmet of salvation; and 6) the sword of the Spirit. The full armor of God is our spiritual defense against Satan's attacks. It's the knowledge that we are acceptable in God's eyes through faith in Jesus. So when Satan tells us we are unworthy, that God could never love us after all we've done, or that God could never forgive us, those accusations will not penetrate the full armor of God. The love of Jesus overcomes his accusations.

The belt of truth is our understanding of the Bible's teaching and our desire to follow it. The breastplate of righteousness pictures the breastplate a soldier would wear to protect his chest in battle. It represents a believer protecting his vital organs with the word of God and his desire to live a godly life. A soldier had to protect his feet in battle. He wore a protective covering over his shoes and nails through the bottom for traction. The gospel of peace for the feet represents gaining traction in our faith and trusting God, which yields peace in our lives.

The shield of faith pictures the small round shield a solider would carry into battle to deflect oncoming blows. Spiritually, the shield represents deflecting Satan's arrows and rejecting any temptation to doubt the truth of God's word and promises. A soldier always wore a helmet into battle. Spiritually, the helmet of salvation refers to our sure knowledge of our own salvation, and therefore our present safety from Satan's attacks. The sword of the Spirit is the only offensive weapon on Paul's list. In battle, a soldier would use a sword to strike his enemy. The spiritual sword is the word of God. When Satan tempted Jesus in the wilderness, three times Jesus parried with him by quoting from Deuteronomy. The sword of the spirit is the word of God, which rebukes Satan and sends him away.

Paul named a final bonus tool in Ephesians 6:18: "With every prayer and request, pray at all times in the Spirit." We have to know our enemy and the tools we have in our toolbox to fight him. Our enemy is Satan, and every believer owns the tools which are effective against him. Whether we want pretty toenails, or success against the schemes of the devil, knowledge is power. Knowing our enemy and how to use the tools in our toolbox to defeat him will get the job done!

CHAPTER 37

PRIDE AND HUMILITY

IF YOU PLAY GOLF, maybe you've experienced this: You and three buddies are standing on the tee box waiting to hit. When it's your turn, you rip one 250 yards right down the middle of the fairway. Your friends spray their tee shots into the woods. You're not very good at golf, but once a round you'll "nut" the perfect tee shot. These are the shots that make you come back to play again. After you've all teed off, you stroll straight down the fairway like a puffed-up rooster while your buddies search for their pathetic drives. Since you're closest to the pin, you're the last to hit your second shot. You stand in the fairway leaning on your 7-iron, looking casually back toward the tee box where your friends are scrambling to get it back in the fairway.

I've done this before but only rarely. The chances of me striping one 250 yards down the middle are slim because I stink at golf. It has happened though. I've taken that walk down the fairway, full of pride over my drive. It usually lasts until I hit that 7-iron into the green-side lake. The pride that I felt quickly dissipated as my second shot reminded me I really stink at golf.

I have a better chance of being struck by lightning than hitting consecutive quality golf shots.

In my road racing the past couple of years, I've taken home a few age-group medals, which is cool, but there also aren't very many runners in my age group. I admit I enjoy winning age group medals, though I wish I didn't. I want to run for the joy of it, to better my own times, and to stay physically fit. Racing for medals is a potential source of pride for me.

It's good to be humbled now and then. On a recent Saturday morning long run, God served me up some humble pie. I was cruising along at my regular training pace, listening to music, enjoying the run, and feeling pretty good about myself. Out of the corner of my eye, I saw a blur pass by me from behind on the other side of the street. She was probably about 40 years old, maybe 5'1" and 100 pounds. I looked down at my watch. I was running about a 9-minute mile pace. Once she was about a block ahead of me, I marked her spot and timed how long it took me to get there. About 30 seconds. She must have been doing something like a 6:00-6:30 pace. It was incredibly humbling.

To make matters worse, as I was recovering from that wound, another runner came up from behind and passed me too. I've seen him many times out on the road. He's at least my age, but I recognize him because he doesn't wear a shirt. Even when it's 20 degrees and I'm wearing three or four layers! He's in shorts, sneakers, and that's it! He blew by me too and any pride I felt about my speed got a smackdown! Immediately, my pace seemed awfully slow. These runners reminded me that though I may beat some of the upper-50's racers, I'm not a fast runner.

I tell these stories about golf and running to show us (especially me) about the foolishness of pride. It's like a cancer that can grow inside us and take over our lives. The potential sources of pride are endless: Golf shots and medals, but money, careers, accomplishments, appearance, awards, compliments, and social status can also cause pride to take root in us. Pride is an ugly human quality. It's taking credit for gifts that God has provided and then acting as if we're superior to others. Pride usually hangs out with his friends: narcissism, arrogance, judgmentalism, and condescension. Nobody wants to be around a prideful person who pumps himself up and puts others down.

The Bible repeatedly warns us about pride. Paul had as much reason for pride as anyone other than Jesus. He wrote in Philippians 3:5-6 about his impeccable credentials as a Pharisee. He was "circumcised the eighth day of the nation of Israel, of the tribe of Benjamin, a Hebrew of Hebrews; as to the Law, a Pharisee; as to zeal, a persecutor of the church; as to the righteousness which is in the Law, found blameless." Paul had every human reason to be proud of his education and accomplishments. After he met the risen Jesus on his way to Damascus in Acts 9, he realized these credentials that formed his identity were worthless compared to knowing Jesus and serving Him.

God humbled Paul and made him see that whatever skills or talent he had were gifts not to be used to exalt himself, but to glorify God and expand His kingdom. To be sure Paul remained humble, God gave him a "thorn in the flesh." In 2 Corinthians 12, Paul said it tormented him and kept him from exalting himself. Although many have speculated, we don't know what the "thorn" was. Paul asked God three times to remove it, but God said, "My grace is sufficient for you."

He allowed it to remain so Paul would never become haughty again. Paul never did. If he ever boasted after meeting Jesus, it was in his weaknesses, not his strengths. Paul constantly deflected praise to God, who accomplished through Paul what he could never have achieved on his own.

. . .

I thank God when He humbles me. When I race, there are always *lots* of people in front of me, so why boast? Whenever I run long distances, I know there will come a point when I'm tapped out, with nothing left in my tank. That's when I pray the hardest for Jesus to give me His strength to help me reach the finish line. It's my body, but His power that gets me there.

Sometimes when I finish, I forget to thank Him for lending me His power! I'm too quick to receive the praise and congratulations of others without giving God the credit. As Paul asked in 1 Corinthians 4:7: "What do you have that you did not receive? And if you did receive it, why do you boast as if you had not received it?" It's a question we should always ask ourselves or pride can dig its nasty roots in us.

CHAPTER 38

BE PREPARED!

I GOT HIT by a car while out running this week, kind of. I came to an intersection with a traffic light and needed to cross the street. The intersection has three lanes in each direction. When the light turned green, I ran across. Before I crossed the second set of three lanes, a car in the left turn only lane sped up to beat the light before it turned red, but then changed his mind. He was about a half a car's length into the intersection and stayed there. Instead of running in front of him, which would have forced me out into the intersection, I ran behind him.

Suddenly, he shifted into reverse and backed up, bumping into my hip. I banged on his trunk with my fist and thankfully; he slammed the brakes. Me against a car in a bumper cars match is no contest. Besides, I have races to run, sermons to preach, and a family to care for. I have no time to rehab a broken leg or hip? My only injury was a rapid heartbeat for the next few blocks. I'm sure the driver had palpitations too.

. . .

My incident reminded me that life is fragile! Some 15-20% of all deaths happen suddenly, without warning. A large percentage of those deaths are by accident, either automobile or other kinds of accident. So often we are stunned to hear of the death of a friend or acquaintance. We think, "How can that be? I just saw him/her the other day!"

We all know death is inevitable unless Jesus returns first. What we don't know is how many days we have left. Whether we live 20, 40 or 100 years, the most important question is what happens after death. We'll all die once. Our first death is physical. Our bodies will die. The Bible describes a second death that is spiritual for those who reject Jesus. The second death is permanent separation from God in hell. These statistics about unexpected death prove that there is no guarantee of tomorrow. The one thing all accidental deaths have in common is that the people didn't expect to die that day. In Jesus' day, people died unexpectedly too. Jesus taught us to be prepared for death by repenting of sin. In Luke 13, Jesus discussed two incidents that were fresh in the minds of His listeners. Some people approached Jesus, asking Him why God would allow Pilate, the Roman governor of Judea, to murder some of the Jews who were offering sacrifices. Their assumption was that they must have earned God's punishment.

Jesus answered, "Do you think that these Galileans were worse sinners than all the other Galileans just because they have suffered this fate? No, I tell you, but unless you repent, you will all likewise perish" (Luke 13:2-3.) Then speaking of 18 people who died by accident when a tower collapsed on them, He said, "Or do you think that those eighteen on whom the tower in Siloam fell and killed them were worse offenders than all the other people who live in Jerusalem? No, I tell you, but unless you repent, you will all likewise perish." (Luke 13:4-5.)

· · ·

The Galileans whom Pilate killed, and the 18 on whom the tower of Siloam fell didn't expect to die that day, but they did. What was the lesson Jesus was teaching? It's not that God was punishing them with death because of their sin. Everyone sins; everyone deserves to die; and eventually everyone will die. Death is part of life. The lesson is that we need to prepare for our deaths by being in good standing with God today through repenting of sin and trusting in Jesus for salvation. Jesus said two times in these verses that God wasn't punishing these people. Death happens. But unless we repent, we "will all likewise perish." By "perish," Jesus didn't mean our physical death, He meant our spiritual death.

That's why the gospel is such good news. We don't have to worry about what happens to us after we die. Revelation 2:11 and 21:6 promise the second death has no power over those who believe in Jesus for salvation. Believers will reign with Jesus forever and ever. I don't think Jesus was trying to "scare" the people into heaven. He was correcting their worldview. They thought they were "good" and that's why God didn't allow Pilate to murder *them*, or the tower to fall on *them*. Jesus was teaching them that no one is good. Everyone deserves God's wrath. Death can come unexpectedly and seem random to those left behind. Jesus said that the wise will prepare!

My run in with a car never threatened my life, but it showed me that death can come suddenly and that I'm no match for a four-thousand-pound car going even 5 miles per hour. Whether I'm running, driving, flying, or even sitting at my desk, my next breath is only by the grace of God. If that car killed me today, it really would have ruined my run! But I've made peace with God by trusting in Jesus for salvation. I'm not afraid of death. I know where I'm going.

A lesson I've learned through this experience is that there is urgency for our friends and family. What kind of friend am I if

I know the way to heaven and don't tell them? If they're not guaranteed tomorrow, how can I let another day pass without sharing the good news with them? Death can come at any moment. James 4:14 says: "For you are just a vapor that appears for a little while, and then vanishes away." At every intersection we approach, there's a driver who *needs* to beat that light! Be prepared!

CHAPTER 39

NOT ALL MILES ARE CREATED EQUAL

A MILE IS 5280 FEET, but not all miles are the same. My last run before a recent Saturday marathon was a two-miler on the previous Thursday. Running only two miles is such a welcome relief after weeks of high mileage training. I enjoyed the run, but it seemed like it was hardly worth the effort. By the time I got into a groove, it was over, and I had barely broken a sweat. By comparison, on marathon Saturday, running two more miles after I had already run 24.2 miles was a whole different story! My legs felt like cinder blocks. My calves cramped and were full of knots. I was deep into what I call the "marathon shuffle." No longer able to lift my legs to stride, I looked more like a penguin than a runner. All this, and I still had two miles to go. There's a big difference between a two-mile run and the last two miles of a marathon.

What about the mental aspect? On Thursday's two-miler I was mentally fresh, happy to enjoy the nice weather, noticing the birds, leaves, flowers, and the signs of spring. Saturday, my mental fatigue nearly exceeded the physical. Long distance running is intensely psychological. Runners must *will* themselves to keep going, step after step, mile after mile, against every fiber in our bodies that are begging us to quit. We play mind games with ourselves every step. "I'll just run to that next intersection, to the next tree, to the next mile marker." We break the remaining distance into bite-sized chunks because after 24 miles, two more miles seems overwhelming and impossible. I pray for Jesus to help me through the last couple of miles, knowing I can't do it in my strength.

Two miles will always be 10,560 feet, but not all two miles are the same. The same is true of our days. There are 24 hours in every day, but not all days are the same. Anxiety or depression can make a day feel like a year. So can grief or fear. I have had a great life. I love my wife and family. My work as a pastor fulfills me spiritually, intellectually, and on every other level. I have a relationship with Jesus, so I know I'm going to heaven when I die. I have no complaints or unmet desires.

My life is great, but not all my days have been great. In 2014 and 2015, I fell into a dark period of anxiety and depression. Between work and financial pressure, the symptoms were so debilitating that I considered even taking my own life. I wrote about this in a book called *Facing Life's Challenges Head On*, so I won't recount the gory details here. Suffice to say, the struggle was real, the length, darkness, and hopelessness of every day seemed unending. What should Christians do when our days are hard and filled with pain?

First, we shouldn't expect that life will be easy. Then hardship won't surprise us. Long-distance runners know what we're getting ourselves into when we register for a marathon. We're signing up for pain, and we're not surprised when it comes. We just need to figure out a way to overcome it. Jesus made plenty of great promises to us, but a trouble-free life wasn't one of them. He said in John 16:33: "In this world you will have trouble, but take heart, I have overcome the world" (NIV.) Pain is part of life as much as it's part of running, so we know what we're getting ourselves into. But the good times and the great runs are worth it!

Second, Jesus didn't leave us without help. Because He overcame the world by His glorious resurrection, and because He sent us His Holy Spirit to comfort us, we can cope with life's challenges too. That's not to say it will be easy, but there is peace available through our faith. Psalm 71:20-21 was a real balm for my soul in my worst days: "You who have shown me many troubles and distresses will revive me again and will bring me up again from the depths of the earth. May You increase my greatness and turn to comfort me." God has promised never to leave us or forsake us even in, and especially in, our darkest days. He will revive us again! It's a promise we can take to the bank. We're not alone even when we feel alone. He is with us.

Third, Jesus taught us to pray. Jesus often spent nights alone in the mountains praying to God. Whatever we are facing, Jesus understands. He lived His entire life knowing that every day brought Him closer to the cross. That's not to minimize our own struggles, but to show us that Jesus identifies with them. Jesus didn't endure life on His own. He asked for strength from God. It's a wise model for us to follow. None of us is strong enough to bear the difficulties of life alone. God never wanted us to. He wants us to commune with Him to get the power we need.

Fourth, remember that God is always good, even though we may not understand His plan. I tell anyone who asks me about my anxiety and depression that God used it for good in more ways that I can even count. That's not to say that I want to experience it again. I don't! But in retrospect, I can see why God allowed me to go through it. I also tell people that though it seems like the pit is so deep that light can't even get in, it will not last forever. When I was going through it, the days seemed endless. The weeks and months dragged on with no end in sight. But eventually, it ended, and it's been behind me for years now.

I was thinking about those dark days during the last two miles of my marathon. Having struggled with anxiety and depression for so long strengthened me to finish. If I could survive endless months of emotional pain, surely, I could waddle through the last two miles. I prayed for God to send a holy tailwind to push me toward the finish line. I asked Him to strengthen my mind for the final push. As I crossed the finish line, I thanked God that though not all miles are the same, and not all days are the same, God is always the same. God is good all the time!

CHAPTER 40

GLORIFYING GOD WITH WHATEVER TALENT YOU HAVE

EXTRAORDINARY MEANS greater than ordinary or different from the norm. God has gifted relatively few with extraordinary ability. There's only one Shakespeare, Jane Austen, Michelangelo, Kipchoge, Serena Williams, Michael Jordan, or Elon Musk. Though the other 99.9% of artists, athletes, and businesspeople lack the singular talent of those prodigies, they can produce outstanding work if they have passion, determination, and grit. By grit, I mean, tenacity, an unconquerable spirit, and an unquenchable desire to succeed.

We runners know all about passion, determination, and grit. Most of us will never win a major marathon. But I have learned, as I'm sure you have, we can overcome a lack of natural talent and ability with passion, determination, grit, and the power of God. God hasn't given me the gift of speed, but He has given me strong will power, and He has taught me to rely on Him for what I lack in talent. Unless everyone else drops out, I'll win none of the races I enter. But unless I die or get seriously injured, I'm going to finish. I doubt I'll ever win a Pulitzer Prize for writing, but I can continue publishing books by committing to typing just a few hundred words a day. Slow and steady doesn't win the race, but it always finishes.

When people ask why I run races or write books, I tell them I do it for enjoyment, and because I like challenges. I like to prove to myself that I can finish races and publish books. But mostly, I run and write because I believe God wants me to. By using my talents, I glorify God. It takes countless hours training alone to get in marathon shape. It's taken me over a year to write this book. Forty separate devotional thoughts inspired by noticing how we can give glory to God by running. I have countless hours invested in it. Will many ever read it? I don't know. A book like this won't appeal to a huge niche. I'm targeting Christian runners. I don't know how many of us there are out there. Since most people aren't Christians or runners, we probably make up a tiny percentage of society. I wanted to write a book that appeals to a unique audience, and that I would want to read. We Christian runners need authors to write books for us too. Though it's taken me *forever* to write it, and few may ever read it, I pray it blesses those who do, and glorifies God at the same time. It's hard to run, and it's hard to write. I have thousands of hours invested in each. But we should all use whatever talent we have, plus passion, determination, grit, and the power of God to glorify Him.

Paul was a man of exceptional passion, determination, and grit. Before he became a Christian, he was a tenacious student, an ambitious Pharisee, and a hardened enemy of Christianity. After he became a Christian, Paul used those same gifts to glorify God. Paul was extremely intelligent, but not physically imposing, or a gifted speaker.

In 2 Corinthians 10:10, Paul was answering critics who challenged his authority. His critics said of Paul, "His letters are weighty and strong, but his personal presence is unimpressive and his speech contemptible." Paul even acknowledged himself that he was not a skilled orator. In 2 Corinthians 11:6, he wrote, "But even if I am unskilled in speech, yet I am not so in knowledge; in fact, in every way we have made this evident to you in all things." Paul did not possess impressive physical stature or outstanding rhetorical speech. He never let those limitations hold him back. He recognized his God-given strengths, intelligence, enthusiasm, persistence, and fearlessness to glorify God. Through passion, sheer determination, grit, and the power of God, he changed the world.

Scholars estimate Paul traveled over 10,000 miles by sea and over land during his missionary journeys in hard conditions. Travel was hard and dangerous, more so for Paul than for others. He was often carrying money to give to people in need, and he had made plenty of enemies by preaching the gospel of Jesus to Jews and gentiles who were hostile to the message. Paul described in 2 Corinthians 11 being beaten, stoned, shipwrecked, exposed, hungry, and in fear of robbers and false believers. What caused Paul to continue day after day? Paul was a very determined person. But he never boasted about anything he did. He always called himself weak and gave glory to God for his accomplishments. He always said it was not him, but God working through him, using the gifts God gave him, that caused the growth of the Christian church.

God can do amazing things through ordinary people like us. Ephesians 2:10 says, "For we are His workmanship, created in Christ Jesus for good works, which God prepared beforehand so that we would walk in them." It inspires me to know that God has prepared things in advance for me to do. I just need to figure out what they are and get after it. The work God has prepared for us will not be easy. We runners know that few things worthwhile are. Thankfully, we're already equipped. God has blessed us with transferable skills. We can use the same persistence, perseverance, determination, and grit we need to finish races to complete the work God has assigned us.

Gritty runners make gritty Christians. What work has God given you to do? If you know, use your God-given grit and determination to overcome obstacles, and keep grinding until the work is done. If you don't know, ask Him how He wants you to advance His kingdom. He's already prepared you and given you the tools you need. We don't need to be Michael Jordan or Michelangelo. We only need the will to serve God with the gifts He has given us. It's God's power working through us that does the work. It's our grittiness and reliance on Him that allows us to continue when we meet seemingly impossible obstacles. My Christian running friends, God can use us if we love Him, and are determined to use the talent we possess to affect people. We might change the world like Paul did. Rely on God to guide you. Use your grit to accomplish His will. God has called me to preach, teach, write, and run for His glory. That's what this book has been about. How can you use your God-given gifts to glorify Him? Ask Him, and then whatever you do, do it for the glory of God!

If you enjoyed this book, I would greatly appreciate it if you would leave a brief review on Amazon. Reviews really help authors because they help persuade others that this book is worthy of their investment. Thank you in advance!

ALSO BY BOB JENNERICH

Get My Free Ebook:

This Is God's Plan?! How We Can Be Certain in Days of Uncertainty

(You can download this book for free by going to my website BobJennerich.com)

Also Available for sale:

Facing Life's Challenges Head On

God Is Everywhere! Recognizing Our Extraordinary God in Ordinary Life

Don't Be A Hypocrite and Other Lessons I'm Still Learning from the Sermon on the Mount

You can connect with me on Facebook at Facebook.com/BobJennerich, and Twitter.com/bob_jennerich. Go to BobJennerich.com find a link to my other books. You can also subscribe to my newsletter at BobJennerich.com. I like to treat my newsletter subscribers well by giving discounts and freebies that I don't make available to the general public. I also like to talk to you! You can also read my blog and listen to sermons I preached at Grace Redeemer Community Church, Garland, TX.

ABOUT THE AUTHOR

Bob Jennerich was a lawyer in a small law firm in New Jersey when he became a Christian. In 2011, he and his wife, Molly, and their two children, Allison and Brian sold their home in New Jersey and moved to Texas so Bob could attend Dallas Theological Seminary. He accepted the call to become Senior Pastor of Grace Redeemer Community Church in Garland, Texas, in July 2017. Every Sunday he preaches the same gospel that he rejected for so many years. He jokes that if you would have told him 20 years ago that he would be pastoring a church in Texas today, he would have thought that you were crazy.

Bob's passion is to read and study the Bible and teach it to others, so that they too may experience the life transformation that happens when people receive the gospel. The inspiration to write books sprung from his passion to spread the gospel beyond the walls of the church he pastors.

Bob also loves to travel and exercise. He's finished 16 marathons. He's a sports fan, but mostly from the bleachers these days. One of his goals is to go to a game in every major league baseball stadium. Only six to go!

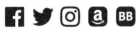

NOTES

1. TRAINING FOR THE BIG DAY

1. https://www.halhigdon.com/training-programs/marathon-training/novice-1-marathon/
2. https://en.wikipedia.org/wiki/Isthmian_Games
3. https://www.verywellfit.com/fitness-use-it-or-lose-it-3120089

2. NEGATIVE SPLITS

1. Bob Buford, *Halftime* (Grand Rapids, MI: Zondervan, 1994)

6. INTROVERTED

1. https://www.dictionary.com/browse/introvert
2. https://www.verywellmind.com/signs-you-are-an-introvert-2795427

9. RUNNING BEFORE SUNRISE

1. C. S. Lewis, *Surprised by Joy*, The Beloved Works of C.S. Lewis, (New York: International Press, 1955), 130.

18. CARBO-LOADING

1. John Tolson and Larry Kreider, *The 4 Priorities: Life is Too Short to Get it Wrong*, (Dallas TX: High Impact Life, 2012), 42-43.

24. RUNNER'S HIGH

1. https://classpass.com/blog/what-does-a-runners-high-feel-like/
2. https://www.roadrunnersports.com/blog/achieve-runners-high

32. MY BEST FAN

1. John Bunyan, *The Pilgrim's Progress,* Edited by Roger Sharrock and J. B. Wharey, (Oxford: Oxford University Press, 1975.)

BIBLIOGRAPHY

Buford, Bob. *Halftime*. Grand Rapids, MI: Zondervan, 1994.

Bunyan, John. *The Pilgrim's Progress*. Edited by Roger Sharrock and J. B. Wharey. Oxford: Oxford University Press, 1975.

Lewis, C. S. *Surprised by Joy*. The Beloved Works of C.S. Lewis, New York: International Press, 1955.

Tolson, John and Kreider, Larry. *The 4 Priorities: Life is Too Short to Get it Wrong*. Dallas TX: High Impact Life, 2012.